Using the Medical Model in Education

Also available from Continuum

Theory of Education, David A. Turner
Theory and Practice of Education, David A. Turner

Using the Medical Model in Education

Can Pills Make You Clever?

David A. Turner

continuum

Continuum International Publishing Group

The Tower Building
11 York Road
London SE1 7NX

80 Maiden Lane
Suite 704
New York NY 10038

www.continuumbooks.com

British Library Cataloguing-in-Publication Data
A catalogue record for this book is available from the British Library.

ISBN: 978-1-44110-427-4 (paperback)

Library of Congress Cataloging-in-Publication Data
Turner, David A.
Using the medical model in education : can pills make you clever? / David A. Turner.
p. cm.
Includes bibliographical references.
ISBN 978-1-44110-427-4 (paperback)
1. Nootropic agents. 2. Education. 3. Intelligence.
4. Neuropsychology. I. Title.

RM334.T87 2009
615′.78—dc22 2009010965

Typeset by Newgen Imaging Systems Pvt Ltd, Chennai, India
Printed and bound in Great Britain by

Contents

Chapter 1

Medical Models in Education

Medical models are widely used in education, and their use is on the increase. Every year growing numbers of young people are diagnosed as having learning disorders, and the treatment is frequently the prescription of drugs. The language of 'diagnosis', 'disorders' and 'treatment' is medical, and we have come to think that the use of these terms is appropriate for the discussion of educational questions. The idea that education is susceptible to medical treatment reaches its height in the concept of cognition enhancing drugs, or 'smart pills'.

There is a great deal of attraction in the idea that one can take a pill and immediately become smarter. In many other walks of life, taking a pill is seen as preferable to engaging seriously with the issues involved – a diet pill is easier than controlling one's food intake or taking exercise, taking a vitamin supplement is easier than eating a balanced diet in the first place, and taking a pill to control an addiction is preferable to exercising willpower. We have pills to wake up, pills to go to sleep and pills to make us happy in the meantime. We should hardly be surprised that young people think that taking pills is a necessary adjunct to enjoying an evening out, or a valuable way of enhancing their academic performance. This is all part of our general and increasing tendency to see all human behaviour in medical terms; learning and thinking are seen as bodily functions. In that sense education is simply the mirror of society.

In this book I will argue that the use of medical paradigms in education is mistaken. I will argue that we accept too readily the idea that learning can be enhanced by medical 'treatments'. But I will also argue that the readiness with which medical models are accepted points to some underlying difficulties in the way that we think about education.

At bottom, the application of medical models in education rests on the belief that the brain and the mind are so intimately linked that an understanding of the brain will completely account for the working of the mind. It is difficult to find the exact language to describe this belief, because it covers a range of positions. Some people believe in a strict sense that the brain and the mind are the same, and that once the brain is fully understood, the mind will hold no mysteries. Others hold to a less rigid, more metaphorical, view, that the brain is analogous to a physical organ, like a muscle, that can be strengthened through exercise. For the time being I have grouped these different views together, because we rarely examine this link between the brain and the mind, so we do not always make it clear exactly which part of the spectrum we are looking at. It has become more or less axiomatic that learning and developing the brain are synonymous.

If anything, this unthinking acceptance of the link between education and the physical development of the brain has become stronger in recent years. Technology has supported this view. Sequencing the genome has made it easier to think in terms of finding specific genes for specific capabilities. Brain scans and images of living brains have made it easier to think that we understand what is happening in the brain when we think. And the development of new pharmacological agents has made it easier to believe that wonderful enhancements of cognition are just around the corner.

In this book I will be arguing that the application of medical models in education depends upon this ready acceptance of the link between the physical and the intellectual. I will further argue that the popular view of a direct link is mistaken, or at the very least requires a much more critical examination. For one thing, the idea that all thinking can be understood in physical terms grossly undervalues the role of the social and the cultural in the development of rounded human beings.

Cognition enhancing drugs exemplify this very well, and will be an important example in my examination of medical models in education. Steroids can help an athlete build up muscle, and by analogy a cognition enhancing drug can make the brain more effective. But the analogy is a poor one, because, even if we admit that a drug can make it possible to think more quickly, or think more (whatever that might mean), there remain serious questions as to whether that would be the same as thinking better, or being smarter, or having ideas that would otherwise have been impossible.

The use of cognition enhancing drugs is the educational topic of the moment. Stories in the academic and popular press are common. On the 16 April 2007 the BBC broadcast a radio programme called *The Defeat of Sleep* (BBC, 2007). This programme presented a range of expert opinion on the use of cognition enhancing drugs – drugs that could be used to control weariness, to focus attention or to improve memory – in a word, drugs that could be taken to make you smarter. The BBC programme was followed, at the space of a few weeks, by a feature the *Times* newspaper (Bee, 2007) presenting very similar materials. And other newspaper articles followed, including one in the *Times Higher Educational Supplement* (Tysome, 2007) describing the use of such drugs by academics. There is a large, and growing, interest in drugs that improve memory, recall and certain mental operations which can be summarized as 'being smarter'.

The newspaper stories covered very similar ground to that covered in the BBC programme. The story in the *Times*, like the radio programme, reported the work of Danielle Turner and her colleagues at the University of Cambridge. She was quoted in the *Times* as saying (of modafinil): 'It seems to improve short term memory, the ability to plan and process information, and helps a person to be less impulsive and more reflective about their decision-making, which lends itself to greater accuracy'.

The high level of interest in the popular media is accompanied by a willingness to take advantage of such drugs. The market for them was estimated to be worth as much as $500 million a year in the USA alone, with as much as half of that being off prescription use (which is to say, the use of those drugs by students and others hoping to improve their performance) (BBC, 2007). The market looks likely to increase. The drugs that are currently being used include ritalin, which has been used in the treatment of Attention Deficit Hyperactivity Disorder (ADHD) for some time, and modafinil, but these seem destined to be joined by a family of drugs developed more specifically for the purpose, the amperkines.

But when I reviewed this material in the press and on the radio I was struck by two outstanding features of the reporting. The first was that commentators seemed to be all too willing to leap to the conclusion that a modest improvement in short-term memory and powers of concentration amounted to 'being smarter'. That is to say, there seems to be a presumption that these pills definitely do work. Commentators started from the assumption that a pill should be able to make people smarter, without much need for further examination. When they should have been asking such questions as, 'Does improving our memory really count as being smarter?', they leapt to the conclusion that pills do make people smarter, and rushed into the ethical questions of whether that would raise new issues of educational inequality.

The second important feature of the reporting was the question of who was thought to be the appropriate expert to comment on the possible action of 'smart drugs'. There were opinions of neurobiologists, animal behaviour specialists, sleep disorder specialists, medical ethicists, psychologists and doctors. Comments from educationists were either rare, or completely absent. It is part of the phenomenon of the widespread acceptance of medical models in education that educationists and teachers are presumed to have no relevant, specialist knowledge when addressing educational issues. I shall be arguing very strongly that this view is mistaken, and that the specialist knowledge of educators is of greater relevance that the knowledge of doctors, neurologists and even psychologists.

These two features of the reporting are, of course, related, and indicate a willingness on the part of general public, and of the popular media on their behalf, to view mental performance as a bodily function like any other. We have seen a distinct, and growing, tendency to see educational failures in medical terms. Doctors, rather than educationists and teachers, are seen as the appropriate experts to talk about, and treat, educational conditions such as ADHD.

The ease with which members of the general public could be drawn in to the notion that 'smart drugs' are possible, indeed available and effective, suggested to me that the belief that the mind could be equated with the brain was an extremely widespread one. And the terms in which the experts discussed the issues involved suggested that they saw the relationship between the mind and the brain as completely unproblematic. Indeed it seemed to me that the idea of smart drugs rested on a rather simple equivalence of mind and brain – a concept that can be described as materialism.

Let us suppose that a person who takes modafinil is able, on average, to remember a 9-digit telephone number, where their normal performance was the ability to remember a 7-digit telephone number. The leap from this to the conclusion that modafinil will make you 'smarter' is so huge as to be nearly unimaginable, were it not the case that this seems to be a step that most people find natural and obvious. We are immersed in a culture where we can all too easily think that we are on the verge of developing an understanding of the inner workings of the brain – and we tend to equate that with the inner workings of the mind.

If the capacity and activity of the mind could be directly related to the activity of the brain, then it makes sense to think that drugs which improve the functioning of the brain will make us smarter. It is fairly easy to think in such physical terms. If the blood supply to the brain could be improved, if the metabolism of brain cells could be increased, if connections between brain cells could be multiplied, then we might be able to think quicker, better and smarter. We would have to put a lot of unanswered questions to one side, such as whether we know how brain activity is linked to thinking, and whether having more connections between brain cells is beneficial, but at a superficial level the argument seems to be compelling for most people. And if most people buy in to the idea that brain activity is good for the mind, then it also makes sense to think of exercise and drugs as appropriate ways of developing the brain/mind in a way that is analogous to the use of weight training or steroids for developing muscles. The examination of the idea of smart drugs, therefore, is an interesting way of examining the underlying values of materialism, and the way in which we think about our own thinking.

The concepts of materialism, and the idea of the brain as some kind of muscle, are very deeply engrained in the popular psyche. Many commentators, and many members of the general public, can leap, without much difficulty, from the notion that taking a pill can help us to remember a telephone number for 10 minutes to the idea that taking a pill could make us geniuses. This leap was often accompanied, in the stories about smart drugs in the popular media, by some very shaky logic, including the argument that 'cognition enhancers' must have a positive effect, or we would not call them 'enhancers'; enhancement necessarily involves improvement. The use of such arguments leaps over a number of important questions, not least of which is whether such optimism was justified. What is it that we believe about education and learning that makes it easy to bridge that gap between laboratory-based tests of recall and the performance of politicians, scientists and philosophers? How do we reach the conclusion that the world would be a better place if only we could remember more phone numbers?

The exploration of that central question, 'What do you have to believe about education in order to assume that these smart pills will work?' is the focus of this book. And in order to explore it, it is necessary to examine the whole question of the link between mental processes and brain processes, a question that has occupied some of the best philosophical thinkers over centuries. Before we move on too quickly to the question of whether we ought to take these pills, we should first examine whether they can do what we seem only too willing to assume. The first lesson that I would want to draw is that the link between the brain and the mind is a complex one, and not to be glossed over quite so quickly. In the rush to get on to what is considered the more interesting question, nobody seems to be asking whether the effects that are reported in the research literature are compatible with the expectations which are being raised for these drugs.

The 'more interesting question' which commentators prefer to address is whether, on the assumption that these pills are effective, it is ethical to take them. And in addressing this question, the most commonly used analogy is with caffeine. If students use coffee and glucose to stay up the night before exams going through their last minute revision, is there any real difference if they take a drug which does much the same, but is more effective?

But long before we get to that question, other concerns should have been addressed. If caffeine is a good analogue for smart pills, then there are a few things about caffeine that we should bear in mind.

I take a lot of caffeine, because I like to drink tea and coffee. I may also be addicted to caffeine. But I do not take caffeine to make me smarter, because I know that the research evidence on the long term effect of caffeine is equivocal at best. It makes me feel more awake, but that seems to be because the absence of caffeine in the system of a coffee addict depresses performance, rather than caffeine increasing performance. After long exposure to coffee in the morning, caffeine simply brings me back to the level that I would have been at had coffee never been discovered.

In any case, I would not be advising my students to stay up the night before an exam doing last minute revision. I know that that kind of learning, which has been described by those who study adult learning as surface learning, is the least effective way of addressing an exam. Immersing oneself in learning over a long period of time, fitting the new learning into one's ways of thinking, and using that learning in developing experience, which has been described as deep learning, is much more effective in the long run. The night before an exam I would be advising my students to go home and get a good night's sleep, confident that they had learned all they needed to for the exam. Or to put it another way, caffeine can be a support, but only for the least effective learning methods. Should we not, perhaps, focus on the ethical question of how 'smart pills' should be described, so as not to give the impression that they can do what they cannot.

Coming back to the question of who are appropriate experts to comment on the use of smart drugs, and what counts as appropriate expertise, we should be seriously concerned by the extension of medical models into the area. In the various popular expositions in the press about cognition enhancing drugs, the opinions of various professionals were presented – psychologists, doctors, neuro-biologists, medical ethicists, pharmacologists. Everybody that you could imagine had an opinion, in fact, except for educationists. Everybody thinks that they understand education without the need for any specialist knowledge. We have all had an education, and therefore believe that we fully understand it.

Our understanding of the phenomena of learning, therefore, suffers a double blow: firstly we assume it is the sort of commonsense activity that can be understood without any specialist knowledge, and secondly, when we feel the need to go beyond the most apparent commonsense, we apply medical models. However, those medical models tend to be applied unreflectively, either because of our faith in the mystique of doctors, or because we do not think that the content of education requires much examination. It is, after all, something that we are all familiar with.

This tendency to view mental processes as though they were physical functions of the brain appears to come to us quite naturally. In fact, this is exactly the assumption that needs most critical examination. If we try to understand learning in medical terms we condemn ourselves to understanding only the most mechanical and least human parts of learning. This is because learning is unlike other bodily functions because the process and content of learning are quite as important as the fact that we learn. A contraction of the muscle is much the same whether we use it to pick up a book or to pick up a gun. The thoughts that inspire those two different movements may look rather similar in mechanical terms, or on the screen of a scan of brain activity. But the content of the thought which inspires those different actions may be very different. Trying to understand learning in physical terms is very like the famous assumption that a Shakespeare play might be written by chimpanzees with typewriters.

In the summer of 2007, the *New Scientist* carried a cover story under the title 'Remote control brains' (Fox, 2007). The essentials of the story were that scientists had managed to genetically modify the neurons of a worm so that the firing of those neurons (and the consequent contraction of a muscle) could be triggered by blue or yellow light. By judicious selection of the neurons which were sensitive to light of each colour, and by flashing light of alternating colours, the scientists were able to make the worm contract first on one side and then on the other.

This may or may not be a giant leap forward for wormkind, but scientists are not shy in pointing to the implications of the development:

> The worm is in the vanguard of a revolution in brain science – the most spectacular application yet of a technology that allows scientists to turn individual brain cells on and off at will. 'It's really

> changing the whole field of neuroscience,' says the worm's developer, neurobiologist Alexander Gottschalk of the University of Frankfurt . . .
>
> 'We'll be able to understand how specific cell types in the brain give rise to fuzzy concepts like hope and motivation,' predicts Karl Deisseroth, a psychiatrist at Stanford University who is spearheading some of the work. (Fox, 2007: 30)

The scientists then went on to speculate that, once they had overcome the small difficulty that the skulls of human beings are opaque, they would be able to stimulate in a human brain small groups of neurons, or even single neurons. Or, in the words of Gottschalk, 'In principle, any behaviour controlled by neurons could be mimicked by turning exactly the right cells on and off using light' (Fox, 2007: 33). And of course, by 'any behaviour controlled by neurons', he means 'any thought, word or deed'.

Now just consider for a moment the hubris involved in that jump from making a worm wriggle to thought control. It involves the idea that we could not simply assert that a thought corresponded to the firing of a neuron in the brain, but that we could identify a particular thought with a particular neuron, presumably on the grounds that the same neuron had the same purpose in every person we encountered. And this in turn would lead to a number of rather puzzling questions: why did our ancestors develop specific neurons millions of years ago? why did they need the neuron that corresponded to the thought of a microwave oven? and, if they had that neuron, why did it take so long for them to invent the microwave oven?

This takes us into realms that have been of interest to philosophers over centuries. One might remember Plato's view that all learning was 'unforgetting', that one was born with an unconscious knowledge of the ideal forms, and one simply needed to be 'reminded' of them through experience. That is extraordinarily similar to the idea that we are born with a brain that is structured for specific thoughts, and we simply have to learn what it is in our environment that those thoughts attach to. But it also means that our early ancestors, who developed this brain that we inherit, had to have brains that would cope with every possible thought that anybody could have now, and in the future. It was a not dissimilar line of thought that lead scholastic philosophers to ponder how many angels could dance on a pinhead.

That is to say, thinking about a mechanistic, physical base for thought in the brain, raises all kinds of philosophical questions that have not been solved despite centuries of concentrated attention. Needless to say, those people who are advocates of the advantages of cognition enhancing drugs are not going out of their way to draw attention to such philosophical difficulties. They would have you believe that the issues are straightforward. Indeed, as one of the contributors to *The Defeat of Sleep* (BBC, 2007) put it, if the outcome of using such drugs was not beneficial, we would not call then 'enhancers'. Enhancement, by definition, represents an improvement. With arguments like that we should not, perhaps, be surprised that the advocates of this brave new world are prepared to disregard two thousand years of philosophy.

In fact, those advocates also overlook the fact that *Brave New World* was a dystopia, not a utopia. Soma, the drug of choice in Huxley's world, was used to keep the populace under control, while rigid classifications of intelligence were used to structure the societal hierarchy. Of course, the use of cognition enhancing drugs does not necessarily imply such a rigid social order. But their use does seem to be linked with a concern over aggressive competition, and the need to ensure that one's nearest and dearest come out ahead in the race to improve intelligence. Thus the principal moral question raised in *The Defeat of Sleep* (BBC, 2007) was not whether it was ethical to give such drugs to young children, but whether it would be ethical to withhold them from one child when other children were using them to advantage in the educational competition for professional advancement. *Brave New World* has undergone a similar transition to the one that has happened to the Midas touch; what started out as a warning and an intended curse has been taken to the bosom of popular culture as a blessing and a desirable goal. It would seem that, in order to sustain our materialist beliefs, we are prepared to recast the warnings that can be found in popular culture to conform to our present views.

Overall, the impression raised by *The Defeat of Sleep* (BBC, 2007) and other similar journalistic reports on the use of cognition enhancing drugs is that in order to believe in their efficacy it is necessary to ignore huge swathes of philosophy and/or popular culture. Without even trying to extend the list that might be involved to Plato or Descartes, it seems that those who advocate or are developing cognition enhancing drugs are blissfully ignorant of the work of Chomsky, Wittgenstein and Popper. That is to say, in order to believe in the efficacy of smart drugs, we need to ignore some of the central problems of twentieth-century philosophy, relating to language, the use of language, and how the development of language is linked to the structure of the brain.

It was these reflections that led me to the central question of this book, 'What would one have to believe about intelligence, in order to be able to believe that taking a pill could increase it?' The fact that we can easily believe in such a pill is an interesting clue to what we actually believe about learning and intelligence. However misguided, the belief that there might be such a smart pill will shape how we address educational issues, and how we think about the process of self-improvement through education. Following that trail is the purpose of this book.

When I discussed this project with a friend, he suggested that I should look at a short story by Daniel Keyes (1959) called *Flowers for Algernon*. The story, written in the first person, describes the development of a janitor of limited intelligence who is the subject of an experiment by doctors who have discovered a miracle operation that will enhance intelligence. The story is a tragedy on two fronts. In the first place, enhanced intelligence does little for the janitor in terms of increasing his satisfaction with life. Initially, it shows him that he is the butt of his workmates' jokes, and that he is not as well liked as he had previously thought. But as his intelligence increases above normal levels, he is also cut off from friendly, social intercourse with anybody at all. Intelligence is presented as the exclusive property of the socially inept.

But the central tragedy of the story is that the hero discovers that he is not the first to undergo this operation. His precursor is the eponymous Algernon, a mouse of prodigious intellect, who has suffered for his increased ability to find cheese in mazes, not only by social isolation, but also by premature death. The implied equation is that a being only has so many thoughts for a lifetime, and once they are exhausted (even when one has run through them too quickly by having a surgically enhanced brain) the being dies.

This story has a number of interesting features that highlight how intelligence is viewed in the popular imagination. In the first place, it is assumed to have a directly physical base which can be subjected to manipulation. Although in the story the manipulation is surgical and in real life it is supposed to be pharmaceutical, the idea that a simple intervention can produce prodigious changes is relatively easy to grasp. The story then presents the resulting heightened intelligence in very negative terms; intelligence is isolating and a social handicap. Presumably, although the image of the intelligent but socially inadequate nerd is widespread, increased mental performance must be seen as positive in real life, or people would not be spending $500 million a year trying to secure it. But one area where the story does signal an improvement over real life is the note of caution, and the understanding that such procedures might have attendant risks.

The risks described in the story may arise from the assumed physical basis of intelligence, and may for that reason be suspect, but nevertheless the idea that there might be risks seems in every way superior to the assumption that is being made by the advocates of modafinil and amperkines, that they are necessarily beneficial and have no adverse side effects. People have generally been conservative about new technologies, and have suggested that the older technologies have in some ways represented a natural limit to human capabilities, as when it was supposed that travelling at speeds greater than 30 miles per hour would crush the body. I would not wish to reject a technology on the grounds that it was new and unknown. However, I do think that perhaps more caution is warranted than is suggested by the claims of Gary Lynch, Professor of Psychiatry and Human Behavior at the University of California at Irvine (BBC, 2007) that we understand everything about these drugs, and there are no negative effects.

Whether or not there are negative physical effects, we need to be on guard against negative psychological effects. Much of what passes as ethical reasoning among those who think that these drugs are a good idea is on a par with the observation that students have always used caffeine to help them with last minute cramming and learning before an examination, and that modafinil performs much the same function, but better. As noted above, those who have studied learning among university students have come to the conclusion that a distinction can be drawn between surface learning and deep learning. Surface learning involves learning by rote, capturing separate items of information, for the specific purpose of passing an exam. Deep learning involves engaging with the material and its contents, and incorporating it into the body of knowledge that one had before, reordering where necessary that basic store of knowledge which one had incorporated into one's world view. And what we know is that surface learning is of little long term benefit, and that most of what is learned is soon forgotten, while deep learning involves the acquisition of knowledge that can be retained much more effectively because it has been appropriately integrated with knowledge developed earlier.

And here we face the real moral dilemma presented by drugs such as modafinil. If they, like caffeine, are effective in promoting what is recognized as the least effective form of learning, should we be promoting them? By admitting the use of such cognition enhancing drugs, are we not promoting the idea that surface learning is good learning, or even the only kind of learning that is important, and that passing an examination by last minute cramming is intelligence. We are in danger of passing on to younger generations a completely misguided notion of what learning is all about, by accepting that drugs might promote it. The one question that was never addressed in *The Defeat of Sleep* (BBC, 2007) was the educational question; do these drugs actually promote or enhance an activity that is educationally desirable?

It may seem odd to ask whether increasing intelligence or improving cognition is an educationally desirable outcome. But perhaps more light can be shone on that question by examining *The Defeat of Sleep* (BBC, 2007) in more detail. The programme packed a great deal into 30 minutes, if not much detail. The opening segment, of about 10 minutes' duration, was devoted to the background to the use of such drugs, particularly in the military. Modafinil had been used by soldiers on active duty to maintain alertness during long periods in action. Soldiers in the first Gulf War used these drugs to maintain their activities while in action for periods of 24, 36 or even 48 hours.

However, the evidence, as described by Greg Belenky of Washington State University in the programme, was that low level mental activity could be maintained for long periods, while high level activity deteriorated dramatically (BBC, 2007). The example given was that the ability to target a moving vehicle was maintained (low level activity), but that the ability to exercise judgement about which vehicles to target deteriorated (high level activity). Between these two performances, there entered a range of possibilities, not the least of which was an increased likelihood of 'friendly fire' incidents, where soldiers could effectively and efficiently fire at the wrong targets. The application of cognition enhancing drugs appears to be effective in producing capable automata, not prudent human beings. If that is not enough to give us pause for thought about what we mean to promote when we 'enhance' cognition, perhaps the next observation of the same contributor should be – namely that among the low level activities that these drugs enhance, performance on standard intelligence tests seems to be included.

As noted above, this was linked to the reports of the work of Danielle Turner. She undertook experiments at Cambridge University on the performance of young, healthy males in some tests of mental agility. After taking modafinil, these subjects found that they could remember a slightly greater number of digits than previously, and could solve simple problems with more assurance. It should perhaps be noted that if the tests were conducted with students of Cambridge University, these may not be typical results. Cambridge University undergraduates will be among that segment of the population that has shown itself to be most capable of managing their own memory and of focusing their attention on problems. I will be returning to this question, the view of education and learning as a process of self-management, as described by Vygotsky, later. At this point I would simply point out that the preparation of Cambridge undergraduates is by no means neutral with regard to the development of self-control in the management of memory and problem solving.

The audience was barely left time to wonder whether learning 9-digit telephone numbers rather than 7-digit telephone numbers was a mark of improved intelligence, before having to face the suggestion, from Lynch, that it was not merely a mark of intelligence, but possibly a mark of genius. The question is a difficult one. Can we imagine what it would be like to be more intelligent than we are? If we really could understand what it would be like to be more intelligent, and to have more profound thoughts, would we not already be more intelligent? What would it be like to have thoughts that were beyond the ordinary?

Lynch's argument was based upon a classic paper in psychology by George A. Miller (1956) entitled, 'The Magic Number 7 Plus or Minus 2'. In that paper Miller argued that people seemed to be able to keep only a limited number of items in active memory, normally between five and nine. The suggestion that Lynch offered us was, effectively, that more is better. If the normal person can hold seven items in their immediate memory, and manipulate them, then might it not be possible for a genius to hold nine things in their mind at one time and manipulate them?

The important point about Miller's original paper is that, unlike Lynch, Miller did not equate being able to memorize seven digits with being able to keep a certain amount of information in mind. To understand this distinction, Miller conducted experiments with subjects who were asked to remember strings of random digits. The result was that they could remember more or less seven, and this result was the same whether they learned the numbers in a binary or in a decimal counting system. But much more information can be coded into seven decimal digits than into seven binary digits. This is presumably why computer engineers (the most likely candidates to think routinely in binary) actually count in hexadecimal, where four binary digits are represented in a single symbol. Miller's conclusion, although apparently not Lynch's, was that this told us something about the way people organized the information they remembered, or in Miller's term, how they 'chunked' it. The novice and the expert would each be able to remember seven things about the topic, but the expert's seven 'chunks' would contain much more information than the novice's.

Revisiting Lynch's argument, having the ability to store only seven items of information in active memory may be a pressing stimulus to reorganize our ideas periodically as we learn, a stimulus which would weigh less heavily on the person who could naturally remember more. Far from being a genius, the person who could simply remember more might be less like a genius than the normal person. The argument might go either way. But we probably need to answer Lynch's original question of whether a better memory necessarily makes a more profound thinker, in the negative.

The idea that we can only hold seven things in active memory at one time may indeed be an important educational idea, and there may be important implications for pedagogy, as developed in cognitive load theory by John Sweller and his colleagues. I shall return to these at greater length in Chapter 5. But the idea that more effective memory is the distinguishing feature between normal people and geniuses seems to me to be the most terrible nonsense.

Some years ago I had a conversation with a friend, then in his late eighties, who complained that he was less able to remember things than he had been in former times. I asked whether he found that frustrating. He answered that he did not really think so, as poor memory was a stimulus to simplicity, and that he found he could think more clearly as a result of poor memory. On that basis, an excess of ability in memory may actually inhibit the reorganization of thoughts along simpler lines and prevent the emergence of genius.

I have no reason to think that he was deluding himself, and suspect that he was correct when he said that the deterioration of his memory was a stimulus to more incisive thought. It would be a rash and immoral step to jump to the conclusion that we should therefore inflict brain damage on people in order to make them smarter. In his case deteriorating memory, linked with worsening sight and hearing, exerted a pressure to be more economical with the resources that he had available. That is a very long way from establishing a necessary link between his circumstances and improved thinking. But in other circumstances we do believe that it is clear what kinds of changes to brain performance will support better thinking.

In order to believe that cognition enhancing drugs can work, one needs to believe that they can have a direct effect upon the physical basis of intelligence. And, of course, for that to happen, one has to believe that intelligence has a physical basis. Brain science, or neurophysiology, appears to offer a key to unlocking this problem. However, although intelligence clearly has a physical basis in one sense, namely in the sense that nobody can think that does not have a brain, the exact link between the operations of the brain and the workings of the mind are less clear, and open to a good deal of interpretation. I therefore saw a study of cognition enhancing drugs as a good way of entering the question of what brain science can tell us about educational processes.

As it happens, two major studies of exactly this question have recently been made, one for the Organisation for Economic Cooperation and Development (OECD), and the other for the Teaching and Learning Research Programme (TLRP) in the UK. The TLRP is funded by the Economic and Social Research Council, and it commissioned a review of what brain science can tell us about educational issues (TLRP, 2007). A similar brief was set for a review of educational implications by the OECD, resulting in the book *Understanding the Brain: The Birth of a Learning Science* (OECD, 2007).

In answer to the question, 'What can brain science tell us about educational processes?' the answer given by both studies appears to be not very much. The OECD study concluded:

> There are few instances where neuroscientific findings, however rich intellectually and promising for the future, can be used categorically to justify specific recommendations for policy or practice. Indeed, one of the messages from this activity . . . is that we should beware of simplistic or reductionist approaches, which may grab the headlines or offer lucrative opportunities but which are a distortion of the knowledge base. (OECD, 2007: 152)

Indeed, the OECD study is anxious to dispel some myths that are based on a supposed understanding of brain science. For example, one of the common extrapolations from brain science to education is based on the physical observation that connections between brain cells seem to increase very rapidly in the early years of a child's life, to be followed by a period when those connections are thinned out

between mind and brain, even on the part of those who are sceptical and critical of specific attempts to link mental functions with brain functions, suggests that promissory materialism is central to the popular view of intelligence and education.

Promissory materialism is really a very strange piece of reasoning. Medical models of intelligence have, in the past, been almost completely ineffective in providing any insight into how the mind works. From phrenology to modern brain scans, very little has been added to what educationists knew about the processes concerned. But for the past hundred years we have been expected to believe that the great breakthrough was just around the corner. There seems to be no more reason to believe that this is true now, any more than it was in the past.

On the contrary, the belief that physical science models will release the secrets of consciousness appears to be based on two quite contradictory principles. The first is that there is a direct physical link between physiology and thought, which is to say that consciousness is essentially physical. This would seem to be the position of the behaviourists, who thought (or think) that one should approach behaviour modification as a scientific question of stimulus and response. Thus if particular nerves are stimulated, particular responses can be anticipated. In that sense, the physical understanding of the brain appears to be quite in line with the project of behaviourism. But on the other hand, behaviourism denies the need to understand consciousness at all. What happens in the mind is a 'black box' with which the researcher need not concern himself/herself. Only the outcome is important.

So, on the one hand, explaining the physical basis of consciousness appears to be a goal which is quite amenable to behaviourist approaches, but on the other it is a goal which behaviourism renders completely pointless. This dilemma will form the basis of Chapter 2 in this book.

In Chapter 3, I will go on to examine the question of what, if anything, is 'hard-wired' into the brain. The expression itself is redolent of the technology of early computers, and the metaphor of the brain as a computer is much, if inconsistently, overworked. In that chapter I will examine the question of whether the computer is a good or poor metaphor for the brain, particularly in relation to language use, and the philosophies of Wittgenstein and Chomsky.

In Chapter 4 I come back to the idea of the brain as a computer, and ask whether anything is, indeed, 'hard-wired' into the structure of the brain. In order to pursue that question it will be necessary to engage with some of the leading philosophers of the twentieth century, Wittgenstein, Chomsky and Popper. Although I tend to the view that there is very little that is hard-wired in the brain, and that anything that might be is relatively unimportant, such conclusions are not necessary to an understanding of the shortcomings of popular expositions on smart drugs and the physical nature of thinking. All that is necessary to put such popular accounts into perspective is the recognition that the question is a vexed one.

In order to develop a fuller understanding of the effect that smart drugs might have on intelligence, it is important to examine exactly what it is that we mean by the concept of 'intelligence'. This is the question that I address in Chapter 4, examining measures of intelligence, including some fairly radical departures from the older traditions of testing such as the work of Gardner on emotional intelligence.

In Chapter 5 I return to the paper by Miller (1956) on the supposed ability of the brain to keep only a limited number of items in active memory at a time. Miller's approach did not lack sophistication, and he was cautious in leaping to any very general conclusions. In both respects he could well serve as a model for his commentators. Exactly why Miller's own arguments undermine a simplistic view of smart drugs, and a possible development of his thought into the field of education, are examined. Again, the result is to highlight the complexity of the issues involved.

In Chapter 6 I present an alternative view of learning, based on the theories of Vygotsky and Mead. Something like a consensus is forming in educational circles that learning is best explained in terms of a theory based on Vygotsky's work, under the general description of 'constructivism'. This will be developed more fully in this chapter to explain, not only why thinking and learning should not be thought of as physical processes, but also why a particular form of constructivism offers a better way of understanding how learning can be improved. This chapter is called 'Attention Deficit', because Vygotsky argued that through a process of conditioning reflexes we can progressively gain increased control over our own thought processes, such as memory and the focusing of our attention. By developing increased self-control over our own mental faculties, we are able to improve the way that we think, implying that the physical nature of the brain does not limit the way that we can think.

Chapter 7 extends the model of learning developed in Chapter 6, to examine its social implications. In particular, I note that society has changed and is still changing in a way that means that the amount of learning required is increasing. Not everybody finds it equally easy to find a place in this new society, and opposition to the new organization is quite natural in those who find it difficult to live and work in this way. Those who are too restless to accept the new order are classified as 'hyperactive'. The consequences of seeing this social problem as a medical one renders it incapable of sensible solution.

Chapter 8 underscores this review of the way in which individuals can take control of their own development and manage it in conscious and productive ways, drawing upon the work of Dweck. Dweck argues that there are two basic positions that people take with regard to their own intelligence; some people think of intelligence as malleable and capable of development through hard work, while others think of it as a fixed attribute like their height or the length of their nose. When faced with challenges, those who believe themselves capable of change and development are normally those who rise to the challenge. There are overtones here of Henry Ford's dictum, 'Whether you think that you can, or that you can't, you are usually right'. However, it is natural that those who think of intelligence as a physical attribute, like height, are more likely to trust physical means of enhancing intelligence, like surgery or drugs.

Chapter 9 examines the 'respect agenda' and the implications of the need for discipline. The concepts of discipline and respect come in two forms – discipline imposed from outside and respect for others contrasts with self-respect and self-discipline. The latter form an integral part of the model of self-control developed by Vygotsky. While externally imposed discipline is important in learning, it is only a stage of development, and cannot be substituted for the whole.

The 'respect agenda' as commonly understood, therefore, represents a freezing of development in an unhelpful way.

In Chapter 10 I look at possible future directions for education, and the implications of the ideas developed in the rest of the book for educational practice. It is paradoxical, though not entirely surprising, that standardization and assembly line approaches have survived longer in education than they have in manufacturing industry. We face a fairly clear choice now between maintaining a system which insists that young people conform, even if that means using the full force of medical science to produce conformity, or radically reorganizing education so that it prepares young people for a world where individualism and choice are guiding principles, and reflection and self-management are cardinal virtues.

Finally, in a concluding chapter, I summarize what has been gained by a critique of the idea that intelligence can be improved through the use of drugs, and recap the main conclusions as to the direction that education should take to promote real improvements in the intelligence of the population.

Popular representations of intelligence and its enhancement rest upon certain medical models of thought and thinking, and of the relationship between thought and brain activity, which are not examined and which seem to be taking an increasing hold over the way educational problems are conceptualized, to the general detriment of education. The assumptions need to be critically examined, particularly in the light of some of the key philosophical frameworks of the twentieth century, namely the developmental psychology of Lev Vygotsky, the scientific philosophy of George Herbert Mead and the linguistic philosophy of Ludwig Wittgenstein. That is to say, the current, popular representations of the educational process require the rejection of the key ideas of the twentieth century and a return to simplistic mind/brain isomorphism.

Popular discussion of educational issues is increasingly dominated by medical models, by the use of pathology as a description for specific learning difficulties, and by recourse to the 'latest findings of neuroscience'. However, when we look at popular accounts of such neuroscience, we find that 'what is now known about the brain' is presented in simplistic and/or downright misleading terms. In addition, educational pronouncements frequently rely on assertions of experts who are working well beyond the area of their specific, scientific expertise.

What is needed is a critical examination of that recent research in order to examine how secure the scientific base is, and how confident we can be when those findings are extended to cover educational settings. For example, drug tests might involve testing subjects' ability to establish new neural networks (as indicated by brain activity in an EMR scanner) when specific drugs are administered. In order to make a legitimate extrapolation to educational behaviour it is necessary to establish that new neural networks can be equated with 'having a new idea' or 'learning', and that the kind of new idea that might be represented by a new neural network can be equated with being 'smarter' or 'more intelligent'. The former question is one that relates to brain/mind connection, a problem that has had a prominent place in Western philosophical thought since the time of Descartes, and is a main line of thinking through the work of Wittgenstein and Chomsky. The latter is similarly a key problem for education, and relates to the concept of intelligence and its formation, which has preoccupied educationists since the time of Binet and Burt, and continues to find development in the work of Gardner and Dweck.

Given the importance and complexity of these key ideas, it seems unwise to assume that biochemists can be relied upon to solve them in their spare time. What is needed is a serious, but accessible, examination of what really is known in the field of science of the brain, and what, if anything, the implications are for education.

Chapter 2

The Physical Basis of Intelligence

This chapter will look at the idea that a particular idea or brain function can be identified with a particular part of the brain or collection of neurons. It will trace the history of this idea from phrenology to its current expression in brain scans and medical reasoning on educational matters.

In order to believe that drugs can improve intelligence, it is necessary to believe that there is a physical basis for thought in brain function. The most obvious candidate for such a physical basis is the idea that memory is based in specific processes, either through the interaction of neurons or through the deposit of chemicals in specific cells. We might call these respectively the electrical and the chemical bases of memory. It has also been suggested that both might be necessary, to account for short term and long term memory respectively. If that were the case, then the efficacy of drugs might be explained by the action of those drugs in facilitating connections between neurons, or sensitizing neurons to impulses, or in their contribution to the synthesis of particular proteins used in laying down memory.

Before getting too carried away with such speculation, however, a word of caution might be valuable. Many years ago, I heard G. E. M. Anscombe talking about the book *Dreaming* by Norman Malcolm. Anscombe claimed not to have read the book, but nevertheless gave a clear exposition of what she thought it was about, namely that dreams do not exist at a particular point in space and time as other events do, but that the only evidence that we have of dreams is the reports of dreamers. As against this view, there is the medical observation that whenever a person is woken in a sleeping phase involving rapid eye movement, they are likely to report a dream. Anscombe argued, as it were on Malcolm's behalf, that if a person truthfully failed to report a dream when they were awoken in those conditions, then we would have to conclude that they were not dreaming. The majority of people, however, argue that they were dreaming, but had failed to remember their dream.

Malcolm's point here is that, if the report of a dream is the sole, reliable proof of its existence, then in the absence of a report we should conclude that it did not happen. There is no doubt at all in my mind that the majority of people have rejected that argument. If I tell people that I never dream, they invariably respond with the argument, indeed the assertion, that I do dream on average eight times a night and that I simply do not recall those dreams. The evidence for that is that most people average eight periods of rapid eye movement per night in sleep, and that this is equated with the number of dream events they experience. In this I simply report what the popular verdict on Malcolm's argument is, without implying anything about its validity as an argument. I have to say that I find it disconcerting that people can, and do, express themselves so forcefully in relation to their belief that they have a better insight into my own experience than I do myself, and that I therefore lean towards Malcolm's view of things, but the matter does not need to be settled definitively in order to see that there is a thorny philosophical problem here.

What is at stake here is a conflict between two contrasting ways of looking at the workings of the human mind, indeed, of looking at the world as a whole. The first, which we might label 'medical', depends upon scientific method as it is generally understood, in the sense that it depends upon external observation of regularities and repeatable experiments. The second, which we might label 'philosophical', depends upon introspection, and argues that reports of one's own consciousness are the most reliable source of evidence about the nature of that consciousness.

Another way of describing this difference in approach is the division between objective and subjective approaches. So, for example, we seem to have two competing ways of describing dreams. The first, which lays some claim to being scientific, claims that observations need to be reliable, and therefore repeatable. The second relies on introspection and self-report, and therefore focuses on the unique nature of the specific experience.

In the former approach, if we wake people up whenever they show signs of rapid eye movement in sleep, and they always report that they were dreaming, then we conclude that rapid eye movement is an external sign that a person is dreaming. In much the same way, if a dog starts in its sleep we might say that it is dreaming of chasing rabbits. But in neither case do we know that that is actually the experience of the person or dog that we are watching; in the absence of a report (which in the case of the dog is a necessary absence) it remains a surmise.

In the latter approach we have an alternative, subjective method of listening to reports of people after they wake up, or of reflecting on our own dreams after we wake up. And this method, of reflecting upon our own consciousness, is the method that philosophers have preferred through the ages.

It should perhaps be added that both Malcolm and Anscombe were students of the philosopher Wittgenstein, and the argument that we must rely on the introspective, philosophical method rather than the supposedly objective scientific method derives from Wittgenstein's discussion of the possibility of a private language, or rather, Wittgenstein's conclusion that such a private language was impossible.

Wittgenstein argued that the nature of language was social. The meaning of a term, therefore, is to be found in the social application of that term. Because of the essentially social nature of language, a method which gives certainty of what a person is thinking or feeling in the absence of a report from them is ruled out. 'I did not dream last night', may be countered by the suggestion, 'You dreamed but you were unaware of it'. But we need to recognize that this is an extraordinary meaning of the term 'you were unaware of it'. 'I called your name while you were reading your book, but you were unaware of it', or 'I stuck a pin in your leg to test your sense of feeling, but you were unaware of it', both make perfectly good sense. But for me to have a dream and be unaware of it, when the only substance that there is to a dream is my awareness of it, makes no sense at all.

However, the fact that we should exercise great care when talking about the internal workings of other people's minds in this way is masked by the fact that we do, in practice, speak in this way, and have invented an entire set of expressions for telling other people what they have been thinking. We say that such events are in their unconscious mind. And by choosing this turn of phrase we hope to gloss over the fact that descriptions of other people's unconscious minds invariably rely on a radical change in the meaning of expressions that we use in everyday language. In everyday language, loving or hating somebody necessarily includes consciousness of one's attitude. Loving or hating someone 'unconsciously' means something quite different, and I am not exactly sure that it means anything like loving or hating as we commonly use the terms.

This question becomes critical if we not only believe that we can find which part of the brain a person uses for a specific function, but actually go looking for it in brain scans. We ask hundreds of people to run over their multiplication tables in their mind while we conduct a brain scan. In every case a particular part of the brain shows heightened activity. We conclude that we have identified the part of the brain that manages multiplication tables. What will we do if we find a person who shows increased activity in that part of the brain, but who denies that they were going over their multiplication tables? Presumably we will say, with the analogy of the rapid eye movement sleep and dreaming, that they were reviewing their multiplication tables 'unconsciously'.

In spite of these difficulties with the objective and scientific approach, generally speaking, we have concluded, as a culture, that objective is better than subjective. The matter is more complex than that, however, as Popper has argued that repeatability is not a valid criterion of either the scientific nature of a statement, nor of its objectivity. The concept of repeatability is linked with the notion, which Popper has also denied, that people learn through the development of 'habits', through the repeated use of specific thought processes. I shall return to this point later, as again this takes us into complex areas of philosophy. I wish simply to note at this point that in most cases a claim of objectivity or to apply a medical model is generally upheld in the court of public opinion.

Medical technology, and especially the technology of brain scans, has so developed that we can for the first time in history have an idea of what is happening inside a living brain. We can, for example, ask somebody to close their eyes and visualize a location with which they are very familiar, at the same time as using a brain scan to see which parts of their brain are more active in the process. Or we might ask them to solve an arithmetical problem or make a decision, and see which part of their brain is most active.

But what should we conclude from such activity? If the person who visualizes a familiar scene is using brain cells in the visual cortex, should we conclude that they are actually seeing it? Or should we conclude that visual memory is in some way linked with seeing? Or should we simply conclude that they are seeing it 'in their mind's eye', a metaphor that we have used for centuries and which all this new technology does little to illuminate? Our natural conclusion is that the new medical knowledge in some way adds some crucial dimension to our understanding, but on further reflection it is hard to see exactly what has been added.

It would, of course, be very interesting indeed, if we could identify exactly that neuron, or tiny group of neurons, that fired when one remembered that two times two is four. But brain scans are very far from being that specific. Indeed, what we know about the activity of the brain from individuals who have suffered accidental brain damage is that if the area which is apparently devoted to a particular activity is lost, the person can, in time, and to a certain extent, compensate by using other areas of the brain. Other evidence, from the brain scans of autistic subjects with exceptional mathematical abilities, suggests that they use different parts of their brain when addressing mathematical problems than the rest of us do (Butterworth, 2001: 11). That is to say, all of the current evidence suggests that it is impossible, and will always be impossible, to identify brain activity in particular brain cells with particular mental functions.

Which brings us back to Malcolm's question, if it were possible to identify the brain cell that was activated when a person recalled that two times two is four, and if we saw in a brain scan that that particular cell had fired, but that the subject reported some different mathematical observation, what would we conclude? Malcolm and I, together with a few philosophers, would conclude that the person knew what they were talking about. We regard a person's report of their own thoughts and thought processes as the primary source of knowledge about those thoughts and processes. The rest of the world, on present evidence, would disagree with us, and conclude that they really thought that two times two was four, but were not consciously aware of it.

On the other hand, we might all think it odd to imagine a classroom of the future, where all the pupils were fitted with personal brain scan equipment, and devoted themselves to the effort to fire their multiplication table brain cells. In learning, we still have the sense that it is the conscious content of the learning that is important, not the physical means by which it is achieved.

In this regard the investigations of Bernstein (1996) are relevant. His studies of blacksmiths indicated that it was not possible to resolve complex human actions into their component parts in a way that is necessary to reduce mind activity to the activity of specific brain cells. Bernstein studied blacksmiths who were capable, because of their skill, in making hammer strokes of precisely repeatable form, thousands of times a day. With a view to understanding the nature of this skill better, he filmed the activity, on the assumption that producing the same hammer stroke could be resolved into a precisely repeatable movement of the shoulder joint, combined with a perfectly controlled movement of the elbow joint and wrist, resulting in a perfectly repeatable movement of the hand. What he actually discovered was that the perfectly repeatable movement of the hammer head was produced by an infinitely variable combination of movements of the shoulder, elbow and wrist. In fact, the only constant in repeated hammer blows was the movement of the hammer head.

Although this study is fairly well known in scientific circles, the implications seem not to have had any impact in the more popular understanding of science, or indeed, in some areas of psychology. Bernstein's studies should have made clear that the project of the behaviourists is completely impossible. It is not possible to build up complex activities from simple atoms of behaviour. Human consciousness controls or apprehends the whole, and will achieve that whole from whatever parts are necessary, even if some of those parts are quite severely constrained. The person who has been trained to receive food by pulling a lever with their right hand will not starve if their right hand is tied behind their back. It is the whole action that has meaning and that is anticipated in intention, not the contributing elements.

We might also reflect on the current movement in education to divide every complex skill into its component parts, or competences. A good teacher, for example, will know how to use different media for effective presentations, how to interrogate a pupil to help them arrive at a logical conclusion, and how to project their voice in order to command attention. One might, as the Teacher Training Agency in the UK has, develop a list of over a hundred such competences that make up the repertoire of the effective teacher. But Bernstein's studies of blacksmiths demonstrate that such a list of competences will not produce a successful teacher; the expert practitioner controls the whole movement, adjusting the elements of that action in order to create the whole, but not necessarily repeating any element exactly.

There is an important development in modern science that is directly relevant here. Over recent years there has been growing interest in complex systems as described by chaos theory or complexity theory. The important feature of complex systems is not simply that they are composed of huge numbers of small elements, or that there are multiple feedback loops through which the elements can influence each other, although these may well be conditions that hold for complex systems. The most important characteristic is that complex systems cannot, in principle, be analysed through breaking them down into their constituent components. The system as a whole, and its sub units, have 'emergent properties' which cannot be understood as merely the sum of the properties of smaller units.

This insight represents a major shift in the basic tenets of the physical sciences, which had traditionally been reductionist in their approach, seeking to describe complex entities in terms of the properties of smaller elements. While some of that tendency towards atomism remains, as may perhaps be the case in the view that it is possible to identify single genes responsible for single aspects of our development, for the most part the science of complex systems is having to come to terms with a more holistic view of systems.

Notwithstanding the general availability of information about the effect that Bernstein described, the contrary imagination, that activities can be broken down into their elements and understood in those terms, seems to dominate popular thinking about how people function. Governments and employers believe that tasks can be broken down into basic units or 'skills', and that if such skills are assembled in appropriate combinations, expert performance will result. Similarly, in the case, which I cited in the first chapter, of scientists who had genetically engineered the neurons of a worm so that its movements could be controlled, no explanation was thought necessary of how this implied that human thought might be controlled in the future; they could rely on us to be able to fill the gap of how tiny elements might be combined to build up a whole that was as complex as one might wish. In the popular imagination, the step from the movement of a worm to art appreciation and mathematical astronomy is deemed to be so small as to be obvious and easily apprehensible.

This desire to break down mental functions into their essential building blocks and associate each with a specific area of brain activity has a long history. In the nineteenth century it took the form of phrenology. According to phrenologists, particular areas of the brain could be associated with particular tendencies, and a measure of how well developed those brain areas were (as indicated by bumps in the skull housing those regions of the brain) could be used as a certain guide to character.

It may seem far-fetched to the modern reader to link recent developments in brain science to phrenology. Phrenology has been consigned to the dustbin of history, along with a number of other discredited theories, such as eugenics, with which it was associated. In the popular mind, therefore, phrenology has been dismissed from our ideas. However, I want to draw attention to the fact that, in so far as it is an attempt to describe mental events in terms of physical events, and to localize specific thoughts to specific parts of the brain, modern brain science is a continuation of the project of phrenology, which suggested that particular faculties and capacities led to (or were produced by) additional development of the brain. Phrenology went further to claim that the skull would show where these areas of particular capability were located. That aspect of phrenology, of reading character by interpreting the shape of the skull, has certainly been discredited. However, the prior principle, that specific mental functions could be located in specific parts of the brain, which is common to both phrenology and modern neuroscience, persists. However, when I first approached that question, I rather thought that the claim that modern brain science was a direct descendant of phrenology was a step too far, and might be difficult to substantiate.

I was surprised, therefore, to find Springer and Deutsch paying tribute to Franz Gall:

> Franz Gall, a German anatomist, was the first to propose that the brain is not a uniform mass and that various mental functions could be localised in different parts of the brain . . . In many scientific circles, Gall was dismissed as a quack on the grounds that there was no good evidence to show that skull shape could be used reliably to predict anything about the person whose head was being measured . . . The basic idea that different functions are controlled by different regions within the brain did attract many followers, however. (Springer and Deutsch, 1985: 8)

The reference to Gall is to the founder of phrenology, and although phrenology is not mentioned itself, there is no doubt that the general direction is described with approval.

If this should still seem far fetched, then perhaps a word of caution from elsewhere would be appropriate:

> There is, though, a more critical reason why the assessment of modern neuropsychology requires some understanding of its history. The evolution of thought about impaired cognitive functions has a remarkably dialectical quality. Just like experimental psychology, but independently of it, neuropsychology became an embryonic science in the second half of the nineteenth century. Very schematically, its history may be divided into four stages, each dominated by particular schools: the rise of the so-called diagram-makers, with their elaborate models of mental machinery (1860–1905); the reaction against them (1905–1940); the switch to group studies (1945–1970); and the development of cognitive neuropsychology (since the late 1960s). If present-day cognitive neuropsychology is to be successful, it must obviously guard adequately against the fatal flaws that were present in the

the structure of the brain. Thus evolutionary psychologists point to the selective pressures that have operated on human beings over millennia. For example, Cosmides and Tooby (1997) give five principles that are the foundation of evolutionary psychology:

1. The brain is a physical system. It functions as a computer with circuits that have evolved to generate behavior that is appropriate to environmental circumstances
2. Neural circuits were designed by natural selection to solve problems that human ancestors faced while evolving into *Homo sapiens*
3. Consciousness is a small portion of the contents and processes of the mind; conscious experience can mislead individuals to believe their thoughts are simpler than they actually are. Most problems experienced as easy to solve are very difficult to solve and are driven and supported by very complicated neural circuitry
4. Different neural circuits are specialized for solving different adaptive problems.
5. Modern skulls house a stone age mind.

Between our ancestor reptiles, ancestor birds or ancestor apes, a good reason for practically any nonsensical reaction can be found – all highly speculative but carrying the apparent stamp of approval of science.

And on the topic of ancestors, why should it be that we now find our ancestry so fascinating? A belief in the physical nature of learning and thinking would make one's ancestry singularly important. An ability to solve arithmetical problems, a tendency to homosexuality, a criminal intention, a gene for playing the piano, almost one's whole life could be mapped out in one's ancestry if only one starts from a belief in the physical nature of the mind. And conversely, a need to 'find one's roots' can only make sense if one has a very strong belief that a great deal of one's way of life is physically determined in this way.

Looking at Chomsky's solution to the problem of induction, he provides a specifically modern, and physical, solution to the problem of induction. A child could not learn by induction the rules of grammar from the sentences they have observed in their short life. But children do seem to learn the grammar of their native tongue very well. As Montessori observed, one learns one's mother tongue without a teacher, and with apparent ease, and one will never learn another language as effectively, no matter how long one lives. For Chomsky, this means there has to be a limited number of possible grammars that one can choose from. To put that another way, the brain is set up so that it can only accommodate a restricted range of grammars, not every possible grammar that one could imagine, and therefore it takes relatively few observed sentences to recognize which grammar the community around the child is using.

Getting from what we can see in specific cases in front of us to general principles is logically impossible, so something must be built into the brain when we are born, so that the selection process is made easier. For Chomsky, this is rules of grammar and syntax, for Hume it is the principles and laws of science, while for Plato it was the ideal types or classifications of language.

The physical basis of this solution to the problem of induction is supposed to be that some connections in the brain are made more easily than others, either as a result of inborn connections or because repeatedly making the same connections makes the process progressively easier. The model which is being held out to us is that learning is the development of habits of thinking, and that habits are formed by repetition.

The question that we have to face here is whether any learning ever takes place by repetition. Popper gives a very clear answer to this question, and his answer is, 'No'. He argues that we learn by making an initial, bold conjecture. In fact he suggests that we learn in this way from a single, one-off instance, and that the removal of such learning, through repeated disappointment with the results, is extremely difficult. He gives, by way of demonstration or illustration, an example from the work of Lorenz, of a goose entering a house (an enclosed space of which it is afraid, simply because it is an enclosed space). On its first entry to the house, the goose follows a path which is not straightforward because it is trying to stay in places that are light (which by implication are closer to the outside). The deviations of its path from the shortest route are removed only slowly and with difficulty. But the initial path was learnt once, on the bird's initial entry to the house, and was never precisely repeated, although features of the initial path were present in vestigial form for a long time after the goose had overcome its initial fear.

A satisfactory physical explanation for memory and learning would appear to depend upon the question of whether one can learn by habit, or by repetition. If we can learn by repetition it would seem to suggest that a physical explanation is possible. But if a one-off Eureka moment is typical of learning, then it would seem that we would need some other way of accounting for learning. So can we ever learn by repetition?

It would look as though the answer is definitely, 'Yes'. You tell me your phone number, and I repeat it to myself several times over until it becomes 'fixed' in my mind. I reach a security door with a friend, and I cannot remember the code to key in, so I ask my friend. I repeat the number a few times to try to imprint it on my memory. It looks as though we can learn things through repetition.

There are two things which need to be said about this, and they are connected. Vygotsky pointed to the fact that, because psychologists base their explanations on simple schema such as this – attaching or conditioning a response to a stimulus through the development of a habit – they are most successful in explaining those of our activities that are most animal-like. Repeating a telephone number in order to learn it may be roughly analogous to the way that dogs learn tricks, through the development of habit. But the second point is that this is not a good way of learning. If, instead of my friend telling me the security code which I then repeat, he tells me that it is the date of the year 10 years after the Act of Union of England and Scotland (and if, in addition, I already knew the date of the Act of Union, and I also knew that my friend is a Scot, and that this is therefore a date which is likely to be significant) I have learned the security code instantly, and without any need for repetition. (And, in case you are wondering, I remember that the Act of Union was 1707, because someone once told me that a seven represented each of the two countries, and that there was nothing in between them.) Learning can happen instantly, and more effectively, if we are able to attach the new learning to what we already knew in a meaningful way. It is those processes, processes that Vygotsky describes as 'higher mental functions', which are less easily explained by physical models.

The idea that the human brain might be 'hard wired' for some specific activities is very common. It arises, at least in part, from our love of the computer as metaphor for understanding the action and function of the brain. But if that is to be our metaphor we ought to see exactly what it implies. For the majority of people the workings of the computer are no less mysterious than the workings of the brain.

The brain has some structures that appear to be committed to specific activities. This notion that there are particular parts of the brain which are hard wired is very old, and dates back to about 1850, when it was discovered that one area of the brain was normally involved in speech. This led in turn to the partially correct inference that specific functions could be identified with particular areas in the brain. In particular, sensory and motor areas of the brain have been identified with some precision.

Importantly, however, most of the operations of the frontal lobes of the cerebral cortex, areas once described as 'silent', do not appear to be identified with particular functions.

If areas associated with particular functions are damaged, as in a stroke, people seem to show a remarkable resilience and capacity for regaining that function using other parts of the brain. Thus while the visual, auditory and motor cortex seems to be closely linked with particular bodily functions, the frontal lobes do not appear to be differentiated in the same way.

The physiology of the cortex has been studied closely, and the cells are arranged in structures that are basically columnar in shape and reach down through the cortex. A single column consists of central neurons, which are presumed to be responsible for transmitting signals to the neurons with which they connect, surrounded by other cells which have maintenance functions, amplifying or damping out the original signal. These various column structures appear to be in competition with each other, increasing their own activity while inhibiting the activity of those around them. It seems that each of the millions of these structures is capable of processing signals, producing outputs which result from a combination of excitatory and inhibitory signals from other groups of neurons.

We might think, extending our metaphor, of the central processor unit of the computer. The central processor unit of a computer is able to deal with those numbers that the computer is currently 'thinking' about, or on which it is currently carrying out specific operations. Typically, the computer is programmed to move four numbers into its active registers, whereupon it can add two numbers together, multiply them or subtract them, and then return the result to memory. Until quite recently computers had a single unit capable of carrying out these operations, although the central processing unit also included a range of fast memory locations so that transfer of numbers into and out of the active registers could be hastened. More recently, as the state of our performance in electronics has advanced, up to four such units have been included in a single central processor unit, making a central processor unit such as the Pentium. This meant that computers could operate a number of different programs in different areas of its capabilities.

More recently still, two or even four of these 'cores' have been included in a single processor chip, giving us dual core and quad core computers.

The important thing to notice here is the numbers. If we think of the columnar structures in the cortex as being analogous in some way to the central processing unit, the brain has millions of them; the most powerful personal computers that we are familiar with have fewer than 20. If this is a successful analogy or metaphor, then we have to expect it to have serious shortcomings as well as providing valuable insights.

We also need to note that the computer is not necessarily 'hard wired'; some of its activities are not located in specific areas of the computer. Although certain areas such as the central processing unit and connections to the peripherals are permanently assigned, memory is allocated on an ad hoc and temporary basis. If I open a word-processing program, the computer allocates it an area of unused memory to operate in. But where that memory is physically in the computer will depend on what else the computer is doing and what other programs the computer is running.

So if we presume that the brain is like a computer, we can be fairly sure that our understanding will at best be partial. And if we further assume that being 'like a computer' implies that each and every function has a specific location where it can happen, and that disabling that area will remove the function, then we will almost certainly be wrong.

Thus, while some functions, and particularly those functions that we share with other animals, such as sensory perception and motion, do appear to be fairly closely tied to specific regions, others, and most notably these include the higher mental functions, appear not to be tied to specific regions of the brain, or at least they appear to be localized in quite large and physically undifferentiated parts of the brain.

The other word of caution about hard wiring is the question of whether this indicates that we are born with certain capacities, or whether we are born with brain structures that are ready to be developed.

For example, as noted above, one specific region of one hemisphere of the brain has been known, for a long time, to be associated with speech. However, in a small number of celebrated cases where children had been deprived of speech and contact with other humans until they were in their early teens, it was found that this area never developed to support speech, and that on learning language those young adults had to adopt other parts of the brain, and that these never developed as fully.

A number of possible conclusions can be drawn from this, among which have been the idea that certain parts of the brain are ready at birth for specific functions, that they need to be applied to develop, and that there are specific windows of opportunity for developing mental capabilities, and that if those opportunities are missed, it will be impossible to compensate fully.

Each of these conclusions is only partially right, however. As the same evidence shows quite clearly, the brain is capable, at least in part, of compensating for the loss of specific areas, so that a one-to-one correspondence of brain area and mental capability is not possible. In addition, the brain develops with use, and interconnections between neurons and growth of brain cells is increased by stimulation. And while there may be windows of opportunity that are important for development, if such widows do exist they are both longer and less rigid than has frequently been supposed. Finally, the ability to pinpoint an area which is associated with a particular mental capability is linked to the kind of capability under discussion; the more animal the capacity, the more likely it is to be strongly localized, while higher mental functions are less likely to be localized.

This brings us back to the general conclusion that the physical functioning of the brain does not determine what and who we are. Recent studies point to what neurobiologists describe as the plasticity of the brain – the ability of the brain structure to grow and change in order to adapt to the kind of thinking that the person is doing. We may know, in a very general way, that people with specific capabilities, such as working with numbers or visualizing spatial relationships, may have particular areas of their brain which seem to be more fully developed. But we still have no idea whether their brain has developed this way because they were developing those capabilities, or whether they have those capabilities because they were born with brains that were better developed in those areas. Nor, and it is important to stress this, are we ever likely to know. What kind of evidence could ever tell us?

This may sound complicated, and it may be attractive to stick with a description that is both simple and appears to offer some insight, such as the notion that the brain is hard wired for certain functions, and that we may hope to discover in the future other capabilities, perhaps all capabilities, that are hard wired. But this question, crudely, is one that has exercised philosophers for several millennia. The mind–body problem, or the question of how our self-conscious, mental activities are linked with our physical activities, is an extremely complex one. A simple answer is likely to be wrong.

The notion that the brain is hard wired is closely associated with a long-standing philosophical position on the mind–body problem, namely that 'thoughts' and 'neuronal impulses' are simply alternative descriptions of the same thing. This position, which is called materialism, suggests that once we know enough about the material workings of the brain, the two ways of talking about what goes on in our heads will be translatable one into the other. We will, on this account, eventually be able to break down complex operations into simple, or atomic, processes, and then see where these are happening at the level of neurons.

For example, when I recognize my mother's face, it is assumed, I have a variety of simple functions – recognizing noses, eyes and ears – and each of these is constructed from simpler functions – recognizing circles, angles, curves and straight lines – and when we know enough we will know which combination of neurons firing in recognition of which combination of curves and lines I recognize as my mother.

Of course, if we think about this for more than a second or two, we are obliged to recognize that it is nonsense for many reasons. Not least of these is that it leaves out of the account the very integrative process that makes that combination the face of my mother. In addition, although I am very familiar with the face of my mother, I have rarely viewed it from exactly the same angle with exactly the same expression. Recognition goes beyond identifying a specific pattern. No amount of laboratory tests recognizing squares and triangles conducted with sleep deprived chimpanzees will actually illuminate what I do when I recognize a face.

The philosopher Karl Popper has argued vehemently against such a materialist view of the mind–body problem. He has also pointed out that there is a pseudo-materialist position, which he describes as 'promissory materialism', which claims that we will be able to adopt a fully materialist position at some point in the future. I would argue that promissory materialism is what much of current brain science is based upon, and I would agree with Popper that it is not a tenable position.

I shall return to these questions later, when discussing how we might move forward in our understanding of education. But for the moment, it is not necessary to come down firmly on one side or the other of this argument. It is simply necessary to recognize that the relationship of the brain to the mind is more complex than can be glossed over in a simple expression such as 'hard wired', or illuminated by a simple metaphor, such as the brain is a computer.

Chapter 4

What is Intelligence?

The question of whether a drug can make a person more intelligent or not, depends rather obviously, on what intelligence is, and how it is conceived. In everyday conversation we have a general meaning of intelligence. We consider the people that we are talking with, how they respond to questions, how they pose questions of their own, how they contribute to the lively flow of ideas, and that subtle chemistry of humour and eye contact that makes them engaging company. And if we enjoy talking with them, we are likely to consider them intelligent.

But such a definition of intelligence is unsatisfactory for two reasons. In the first place it is vague and impressionistic. I judge that one child is more intelligent than another purely because I form a subjective impression, and another person might well not agree with me. Parents are notoriously likely to think that their child is more intelligent than any other, and personal bias, willingness to interpret a response as intelligent, and familiarity may all influence the judgement. The apocryphal story is told of a child taking an intelligence test, who was confronted with the question: Take 9 away from 93 as many times as you can; what is your answer? The child wrote down, 'I make it 84 every time'. Whether that is an extremely intelligent response or an extremely foolish one is likely to depend upon the judgement of the observer.

The other problem with intelligence judged as the ability to be an engaging party to a conversation is that it depends very strongly on the situation. A person who sparkles with intelligence and wit in a conversation about fishing may have almost nothing to contribute to a conversation on family history, or better things to do than to engage in it in the first place. And our wish is to see intelligence as a characteristic or trait of the person, not of the conversation that they are involved in.

At the beginning of the twentieth century, psychologists started to look to overcome the first of these difficulties by developing standardized intelligence tests. These were designed to measure mental ability, and to assign it a number which was valid and reliable, normally expressed as an intelligence quotient or IQ. The advantage of expressing the score as IQ, if it is an advantage, is that IQ can be seen as invariant with age. It is reasonable to expect, if we take an intelligence test, that a 14-year-old will get more questions right than an 11-year-old (on average). But by expressing intelligence with reference to the average performance of people of the same age, an 11-year-old who has average performance on the test will be given the same score as an average 14-year-old. In fact both will have an IQ of 100, because, by definition, the average IQ of any age cohort is 100.

Intelligence tests, therefore, are standardized so that when a particular cohort of people take the test, the scores on the test are distributed so that the mean score is 100 and the standard deviation of the distribution is 15. In general terms, that means that almost everybody taking the test will have an IQ between 55 and 145, and that about half the people will have an IQ between 85 and 115. The fact that an IQ test produces a consistent distribution, and that an individual's score remains constant, within fairly narrow limits, assures the reliability of the test. In fact, that is what we mean by the reliability. At some level, we know that a person's performance on an intelligence test will not always give the same result. People have off-days. They practise. They have 'eureka moments' where they realize what a particular type of question is about. But our view that intelligence is a characteristic of the person involved means that we are prepared to accept IQ as being a more or less adequate measurement of some underlying property of the person which does not change, or does not change very much.

As to the validity of the intelligence test, this rests upon the idea that it measures what it is supposed to measure, that a person who has a high score on an intelligence test is actually intelligent. And this is a difficulty, because we all know people who have high IQs, but who are not only poor conversationalists, but who are remarkably stupid on a whole range of other, impressionistic criteria. Similarly, we know people with low IQs who are both thoughtful and show wisdom beyond their IQs. The idea of somebody who is extremely intelligent but who lacks street-smarts, and vice versa, is the stuff of jokes and situation comedies. At some level we are quite familiar with the notion that intelligence tests are very far from valid.

However, the search for reliability and validity, or to put it another way, the search for some measure of scientific credibility, means that it could not really be acceptable to live with a situation where intelligence tests were seen as lacking in either. The idea has become increasingly embedded in our way of thinking over the last hundred years that intelligence is what intelligence tests measure. While, informally, we are prepared to accept that a geek is somebody with prodigious mental capacities and poor social skills, formally, IQ and intelligence have become inextricably linked as concepts. In that sense, the validity of IQ tests has been resolved by definition, and all that one would need to do to ensure the validity of a new test is to show that it correlated well with earlier tests. But the reliability of IQ tests produces other, different problems.

Once we are in possession of IQ tests, it seems that we should be able to address a lot of interesting questions, such as whether people have become more intelligent over the last 100 years. We could take a test from the 1940s and give it to children today, and see whether children did better on it today than they did then. In fact, it is well established that scores on intelligence tests have risen consistently over time (Flynn, 2007). Unfortunately, we are caught in a cleft stick here. If we accept that IQ is rising over time, we undermine the reliability of the tests, since these are supposed to be reliable, and hence repeatable. On the other hand, if we say that IQ is invariant, we will have to standardize the old test on the new generation, and we will be obliged, by definition, to come to the conclusion that the average IQ of children now is, as it has always been, 100. And this, of course, means that we cannot address the question of whether intelligence has risen in the last 100 years.

A similar problem arises in relation to the comparison of different groups. If the test has been standardized on North American or European children from middle class backgrounds, as most of the early tests were, then they could not easily, or legitimately, be applied to other groups. On the other hand, if they had been standardized on a wider range of children, they could say less about the differences between different groups of children. Even so, it would be possible to imagine a test which was standardized on a mixed group of children, but which nevertheless gave different scores for different groups. Consider, for example, a test that had been standardized as having a mean of 100 and a standard deviation of 15 on a group population of boys and girls, but which nevertheless gave different distributions for boys and girls. We might, for example, imagine that girls had a mean of 105, while boys had a mean of 95. This would necessarily mean that there was something in the test, some items in the test, that girls found easier than boys did. ('Found easier' is itself a rather telling expression. It could, of course, be that the girls had worked harder at a particular aspect of the test, or found something in the experience of their gender that meant they were better prepared for some items, but because they did better, we say that they 'found it easier'.)

Generally speaking, the response to this difficulty has been to remove such items, on the grounds that those items indicated cultural bias in the test, and that the items were therefore not appropriate to an intelligence test. We have seen, over time, a winnowing out of items until intelligence tests consist of a narrow range of elements which are culturally neutral, our ability to answer them is roughly constant over time, and for which no special training or preparation provides an advantage. In short, we think that we have found tests which measure a capacity of the individual in relation to their mental abilities, which is more or less constant through life, and is relatively unaffected by any educational experiences.

We are all familiar with the kind of tests that result from this winnowing process – arithmetic, verbal reasoning and logical patterns are pretty much the only test items which remain in intelligence tests. The result is something like reliability; any population, and pretty much any easily identifiable sub-population, will have a mean of 100 and a standard deviation of 15. This has now reached the point where that property alone is almost enough to define an intelligence test. But the 'better' intelligence tests have become, the less interesting they have become.

Ask whether Americans or Australians are more intelligent, and administer an intelligence test to a sample of both populations, and any difference between the two probably arises from the fact that the test has been standardized in only one country. If the test has been standardized on samples from both countries, any difference between the two countries can probably be accounted for by cultural bias in the test. The external validity of intelligence tests has virtually disappeared, and it is now true to say that intelligence tests measure very little apart from the ability to answer intelligence tests. And, in spite of a great deal of ink and paper that has been wasted on heated debates, intelligence tests are not capable of telling us much about the differences between different groups of people either.

Interestingly, *The Defeat of Sleep* (BBC, 2007), the radio programme that set me thinking about the question of smart drugs in the first place, noted that drugs such as modafinil seemed to enhance the performance of low level skills, such as recall from memory or carrying out routine operations, but did not enhance higher level skills where the exercise of judgement was necessary. And among those lower level skills that were enhanced, performance on intelligence tests was included. This is an interesting, and not particularly positive, evaluation of where we now stand in relation to the concept of intelligence.

In parallel with the development of intelligence tests, an alternative view of mental capabilities was developed, which saw intelligence as a hierarchy of skills. This view, most clearly expressed in Bloom's Taxonomy (Bloom, 1956), described a range of abilities from simple recall, through analysis and synthesis, to application and problem solving. While this confirms the view that the things that intelligence tests (and academic tests and examinations more widely) measure have a distinct tendency to be at the lower end of the hierarchy, it makes it much more difficult to conceive of intelligence as a single characteristic of a person. More importantly, it makes it clear that one can develop the higher levels of intelligence through a process of education.

Particularly in relation to higher mental functions, Vygotsky pointed out how social and cultural tools could be incorporated into our natural or lower mental functions in order to augment them. He described this in relation to memory. Children of different ages engaged with an exercise in which they were given a series of questions, the answer to each of which was a colour word. They were not allowed to use the same response twice. In order to help them develop their skills in this task, Vygotsky provided a set of cards, each with a different colour word on it. Children were shown how they could use the cards as prompts, to remind them which words had already been used (Rieber, 1997: 154–6).

Children of 4 and 5 found the cards not to be helpful; they responded to the questions spontaneously, without thinking to use the cards to support their answers. But children of 5 and 6 used the cards effectively to improve their performance. However, this advantage provided by the cards diminished with time as the children internalized the process and managed to respond accurately without use of the card. Similarly, older children, who had already internalized methods of managing their memory, found the cards not to be useful at all.

Vygotsky argues that it is through this process of incorporating social symbolic systems to improve the management of our own internal mental functions that we can progressively improve. It took untold ages of developing arithmetic for society to decide upon the usefulness of the decimal point and the notation of numbers where place indicates value. At first, each of us learnt this through drills and exercises in our schools, but we have gradually so incorporated it into our thinking that we do not need to make conscious reference to it; when we see a number we know that the digits are given values according to their positions.

Vygotsky drew a distinction, in the case of memory, between mnemonic processes (those which were the capabilities of the unaided memory) and mnemono-technical processes (in which the native functions of memory are supported by the use of techniques and symbolic schema that have been incorporated from the social world). Needless to say, for anybody who has lived for more than a few years, all mental processes become a complex hybrid of the two, or to describe this in another way, the mnemonic processes, processes that we think of as 'natural', become extended and more complex, and therefore more capable of incorporating the next mnemono-technical improvement. Vygotsky also pointed out that the advantage produced by a mnemono-technical method – the difference in performance between the aided and the unaided memory – gradually diminishes as the method becomes more fully integrated into the mental processes of the person. Once the children had learned how to use the cards, it soon became clear that they did not need the cards as they were able to manage their memory without them. However, he went on to suggest that this law of diminishing returns was a feature of the laboratory situation, and that in a broader social context, if technical support for memory, for concentration, for focusing attention and for all the other higher mental functions was continuously provided, the performance of the brain could be continuously and indefinitely improved (Rieber, 1997: 186).

This is quite a different view of intelligence from that which is measured by intelligence tests. It suggests that my intelligence is no longer something which is entirely contained within my brain, but that it extends to, and is extended by, those tools that I use for managing knowledge – the computer spreadsheets and databases, the library card indexes and catalogues, the abstracting services and the Internet discussion groups. Some part of those things has been incorporated into my way of thinking, and that makes the rest, or much of the rest, readily accessible.

But this notion of intelligence highlights the shortcomings of the concept of intelligence that can be measured with an intelligence test and assigned a score. These are mental functions that change (and improve) over time, and which are very strongly influenced by past experiences. It is an account of intelligence as it relates to everyday life rather than to the academic world. If I want to know whether somebody is a good architect, I would generally judge that by looking at work that he or she had done before, work done with full access to works of reference, computational aids, consultation with colleagues, whatever it takes to get the job done. But we continue to place a very high degree of trust in artificial tests of ability, performance in timed examinations with no access to reference texts, to computational aids, and certainly not discussion with colleagues.

Increasingly, academics in higher education are coming to terms with this discrepancy. The literature refers to deep learning and surface learning. Deep learning is the kind of situated learning that draws upon resources, internalized mental schema and personal development of higher mental functions. Surface learning is learning for the test, relying on short term recall and the limited development of higher mental functions. And it is generally agreed that the self-management and self-regulation that is implied in deep learning makes it preferable to surface learning.

So why is the earlier notion of intelligence, as a personality trait which does not change over time, so firmly entrenched in our way of thinking, and therefore in our educational system? I think that there are two answers to this question. The first relates to academic disciplines and the organization of knowledge. As Vygotsky noted, psychology has been most successful when dealing with the lower mental functions, when dealing with those aspects of our mental lives that can be easily quantified and correlated (Rieber, 1997: 37). Educational psychology has developed almost entirely on the basis of tests that are valid and reliable. That is to say, intelligence tests have bolstered the development of educational psychology, and the focus of educational psychology has been on the measurement and study of the lower mental functions that could be captured in this way. (The situation would seem, at long last, to be changing now, with some welcome developments in social psychology, and the work of educationists such as Dweck (1999).)

But the other concern that relates to intelligence testing is an issue of social justice. We have in the past aspired to provide higher levels of education to all who can benefit from it at the point of entry. Thus, when secondary schools were competitive (if that can be put in the past tense), we wanted to admit the most able children to grammar schools, irrespective of the social position of their parents. Similarly, we want to provide higher education for all who deserve it, providing bursaries to those who cannot afford it, so that all societal groups can benefit equally. The problem of social justice which we face is that parents can buy advantage if we test for admission using an examination the outcome of which can be influenced by experience. We prefer to ignore it, but any state subsidy of higher education tends to go, on average, to the wealthiest social classes, because wealthy parents can secure better secondary education for their children, and are therefore disproportionately represented among the intake to higher education.

We would prefer to have a measure of intelligence which was not affected by the previous educational experience that the young person has had. If such a test were possible, then we would be able to admit the most intelligent 50 per cent of the population to universities, and that 50 per cent could be drawn from the whole population irrespective of wealth or background. We would like neutral tests of 'scholastic aptitude' or intelligence, which do not depend upon previous experience, and which would be capable of solving this social justice conundrum for us.

Needless to say, this is complete nonsense. In practice we know, as Vygotsky knew, that previous experience can help us to develop and internalize ways of thinking, systems of symbolic representation and techniques of self-management which improve our higher mental functions. What we can learn next depends upon what we have learnt before. And our ability to benefit from higher education depends very much on the secondary education we have experienced. But resolving our problem of social equity will require very much more radical and more imaginative solutions if we admit this obvious truth.

In his incisive critique of the way modern media are affecting education, Postman (1985) notes that successful, long-running television series are designed so that a member of the audience can dip into a single episode without needing to know what has happened in previous episodes. It would be economically ruinous to insist that the plot of a situation comedy should run through all the episodes in the way that the plot runs through a novel. To do so would mean that an established series could not attract a new audience, and in ratings wars, 'inclusion' is more important than anything else. Postman's point is that in education we are now moving the same way, by modularizing curricula and playing down the need to develop some mental capabilities before others can be developed.

We know that it would be complete foolishness to ban mathematics classes from secondary school so that all young people could compete on a level playing field for places to study mathematics at university. But still we try to maintain the idea that measures of intelligence can in some way permit us to be equitable, and to overcome the difficulty that some children have had richer early experience than others.

Before moving away from this review of the concept of intelligence, there are some other developments of the concept which should perhaps be mentioned. Piaget became involved in the question of mental development in young children through his work with intelligence tests. Unlike most of those who have worked in this field, Piaget became interested in the wrong answers that children gave rather than the right ones. He observed that the wrong answers were characteristic of the child's stage of development, and that children would be distracted by different wrong answers as they developed. From this he deduced a theory of mental development, which suggests that children go through different, distinct stages of mental development, in each of which their thought processes are quite different.

This has a number of definite advantages over the view that intelligence is constant throughout life, as it does incorporate the idea that the child is using his or her engagement with the environment to develop thinking and understanding. However, Piaget's theory is most commonly linked to a developmental model which implies that mental developments are largely maturational, and depend upon the development of the brain through ageing and growth. That is to say, Piaget was more interested in identifying which mental processes were being used by a child, than in studying how they developed, or how they could be promoted. Consequently, text books that describe Piaget's model of development have a tendency to describe the stages of development of the child as being attached to certain age groups. The evidence to support this from brain science is poor, and in general the model gives teachers and parents very little guidance on how to support a child in the move from one stage to the next. For both of these reasons, Piaget's model seems to me to be inferior to the insight offered by Vygotsky.

Even among those psychologists and educational testers who took the view that intelligence is constant throughout life there have been debates and controversy. One of the major ongoing discussions has been the question of whether intelligence is one thing or many. Is there one general characteristic which can be described as general intelligence, and which determines how successful one will be in all spheres of intellectual endeavour, or are we blessed with mathematical intelligence, language intelligence, aesthetic intelligence, and many other specific forms of intelligence in addition to general intelligence?

At the heart of any debate such as this there is a difference over statistical methods. Those who believe that there are multiple intelligences think that the correct way to proceed is to apply factor analysis to the items used in intelligence tests, and demonstrate that facility in some questions is correlated with facility in others. In this way it is possible to separate groups who do well or poorly on this group of questions or that. This evidence for different factors or different forms of intelligence will be seen by others, however, as suggesting that these items are not measuring intelligence at all, and should be excluded from the test. As ever, statistical methods can be used to buttress the position which one wishes to adopt anyway, and the reader can choose whether to believe that intelligence is single or multiple as they please.

Again, I think there is a sense of social equity involved in the notion of different kinds of intelligence. We like to believe that there is some kind of fairness in the world, and that those who lack the kind of intelligence that is valued in schools have the benefit of some other kind of intelligence that relates to handicraft or sports or something else. This is a reassuring notion, but so at odds with anything that I have ever seen in a classroom that I think it has little purpose but to justify the exclusion of some people from education, on the grounds that they have other, different talents. I think that is another area of concern which might be considered when we do take issues of social justice seriously.

The latest addition to the range of multiple intelligences on offer is emotional intelligence. The idea behind this is that some people are certainly very clever in terms of their IQ, but they are obviously self-destructive in other ways. To be successful, one has not only to be intelligent, but also to be able to express oneself emotionally, to manage oneself in a responsible and open way, and not be so needy that one falls into the traps which await the intelligent, from addiction to obsession. I think that many educationists see emotional intelligence as a useful concept to broaden the general concept of intelligence, and to provide a counterbalance to an idea of intelligence that is purely intellectual and based on logic and verbal reasoning. For me, on balance, it is a negative idea, in the sense that it stands to contaminate our understanding of emotions with all the wrong-headedness of intelligence, and is likely to lead to the view that emotional capability is fixed for life, does not depend upon experience, and can be measured in a simple test.

Finally, coming back to the question of drugs which can enhance mental capacity, one can imagine physical conditions which might improve mnemonic memory and other higher mental functions (concentration, reflection and so on). Good food and plenty of rest might make the brain cells more capable of discharging their functions, and memory and concentration might be improved. And we might think of a drug that could help in maintaining that condition.

Those of us who are addicted to caffeine might even argue that we have found one. The research suggests otherwise, but that does not stop me thinking that a good strong cup of coffee in the morning helps me to think better at work in the morning. The research suggests, rather, that long term use of caffeine actually depresses the normal level of performance of the mind, and that the boost that a strong cup of coffee gives does no more than bring me back to the level that non-coffee drinkers manage to attain normally (James et al., 2005). But it has been suggested that cognition enhancing drugs are the moral equivalent of caffeine. For example, article in the *Times Higher Education Supplement* (Tysome, 2007) cites the opinion of a researcher in bioethics as saying, 'These drugs might, at the very least, be an improvement on caffeine, the current mental stimulant of choice for many students and academics'. The report of the Academy of Medical Sciences (2008: 158) implied a similar equivalence, while noting elsewhere (ibid.: 149) that the general public drew a distinction between cognition enhancing drugs and caffeine, on the basis of their long familiarity with the latter. Consequently, it might be fruitful to follow the analogy between cognition enhancing drugs and caffeine a little further.

Who has not, after all, sat up late revising for an exam, fuelled on sugar and caffeine, in order to cram in the last few items of knowledge, content in the understanding that once the exam is over those pieces of information will pass from the memory as though they had never been present? In short, caffeine is used as a support in surface learning, in the development of the form of intelligence which is acknowledged to be of least use, and in activities which do least to develop or measure higher mental functions.

I certainly use drugs to manage my own motivation. My drugs of choice are coffee and chocolate. When I face a chore, such as reading through a large number of student assignments, I divide it up into quarter or half hour stretches, and place breaks with incentives at appropriate points, in order to ensure that I concentrate properly on the chore. But there is a world of difference between using what one knows about oneself to manage one's own behaviour, and expecting that taking a pill will do all of that automatically. So what we need to recognize in evaluating the possibility of a smart drug is that drugs may enhance mental performance in some aspects and in some conditions, but that generally speaking they support the functions that are least valuable to personal and professional development. Our moral obligations stretch to making this clear to those who might be tempted to use such drugs.

The size of this task should not be underestimated. Consider the claim made by the evolutionary psychologists, that the modern skull houses a stone age mind (Cosmides and Tooby, 1997). If we take a rigorously non-materialist perspective, then we have to see that the modern skull not only houses a modern mind, but that the modern mind is much better than the mind of 10,000 years ago, or even 50 years ago.

I cannot speak for you, but my modern mind is furnished with a range of cultural tools which have become available at very specific historical points in time. I can count using a number system that uses place value and the symbol for zero, my understanding of my place in the cosmos is informed by the work of Copernicus, I can understand differential calculus, I use a watch and diary to manage my social obligations, and I know how to use a computer to communicate with other people, analyse data and manage information.

In evolutionary terms, my brain is a stone age brain – or a modern brain if you wish, as evolutionary changes are so slow that there is no difference. But that does not mean that I am condemned to having a stone age mind. My mind, like yours, is stuffed with modern ways of understanding and thinking, and modern tools for organizing perceptions. Of course, we were not born with them, and we have incorporated most of them so firmly into our ways of thinking that we think that they are 'natural'. But that should not blind us to the fact that most of the tools that we use for managing our thinking would not have been available even a few generations ago.

Nor are those tools for managing our performance equally available to everybody. People in industrialized societies routinely use symbols to manage their performance and interactions. In fact, they use them so routinely that they have almost disappeared from our consciousness. When the hour glass appears on the screen of the computer, I know to take a pause for thought and breath, because the computer is not going to respond to anything that I do. I do not even think about the complexity of social organization that I accept when I see a road sign that tells me which way to turn. Symbols such as these for organizing ourselves are ubiquitous, and so routine that they have become invisible.

Some years ago I visited a project in rural education in Mexico. One of the lessons which the project was trying to convey was this ubiquity of symbols in managing human affairs. But, and this struck me very forcefully, in Mexican rural communities such symbols are not ubiquitous. One tutor pointed out to us that in order to find such a symbol, the nearest road sign, members of the community had to walk for over half an hour. The cultural furniture of minds is not evenly distributed among people, and increasing fairness in its distribution is the function of education.

Perhaps I should add a comment, about the values that I employ here. I have argued that the modern mind is different from the stone age mind. But more than that, I have argued that the modern mind is better. This does not mean that I accept that all scientific development is 'progress', or that all change is for the better. There is no particular virtue in being able to recite the alphabet or chant one's seven times table. Such things can be used as much for oppression as for liberation. I might as easily have talked about advertising hoardings for casinos and alcohol as about road signs, and I would not necessarily regard those elements of modern society as much better than the way our ancestors arranged their lives. But when these things acquire positive value is when we use them, consciously and reflectively, to organize our own thinking and manage ourselves. We create ourselves through the range of mental furniture we choose to incorporate into ourselves. And we currently have a much larger, and growing, range of tools for self-management available to us than any previous generation.

I have set out here a view of human intellectual development which is based upon the views of Vygotsky, Dewey and Popper. There is a contrasting view of human intellectual development, or perhaps the lack of it, which is based on the views of Darwin and Hobbes, that life is 'nasty, brutish and short'. I do not have any great argument with Darwin and Hobbes when it comes to explaining the organization of our brain, or the workings of our lower mental functions. What I argue is that the culture and learning that we build on our animal foundation is more important, and capable of over-riding our genetic inheritance. But it appears much easier for most people to believe that our minds are primitive, and that our experience, both personal and cultural, does not add anything substantial to the way we function. And it is the gap between these two approaches that is a measure of the task that we have to come to terms with in managing our non-material selves.

In summary, our view of intelligence has become inextricably linked with our efforts to measure it. For reasons that had a positive motivation in the first place, such as instilling our concept of intelligence with scientific reliability, or finding measures of intelligence that will help us to ensure that access to education is provided on a fair basis, we have designed intelligence tests in specific ways. Such approaches to intelligence are tied in with our other views on education, such as the question of whether the learner is responsible for their own learning, or whether learning is the outcome of being put in situations which are beyond his or her control. I have written elsewhere about those more general issues of modelling the educational process, and pointed to what I think are the shortcomings of the normal way of thinking about causation in education (Turner, 2004 and 2007). But what needs to be borne in mind in relation to the possibility of smart drugs is that our commonsense view of intelligence is infused with our commonsense views of both science and education, and those views incline us to think that smart drugs will increase intelligence in an unproblematic way. If we think of education as something which is 'done' to young people, and that knowledge is 'transmitted' from the teacher to the learner, it is natural to think of intelligence being improved by something that improves physical channels of communication. If our commonsense concepts of intelligence and education are flawed, as I believe they are, the idea of smart drugs will be much more complicated.

Chapter 5

Thinking Harder or Thinking Smarter?

In the *Defeat of Sleep* (BBC, 2007), Professor Gary Lynch of the University of California at Irvine tries to give an illustration of what it might mean to visualize being smarter. This is an interesting question which appears very straightforward. After all, if it really is possible to imagine that taking a 'smart drug' will make one more intelligent, it ought to be possible to apprehend, just as easily, what being smarter would be like. If I want to be smarter, what, exactly, is it that I want to be able to do that I cannot do now?

Lynch offers what, on the face of it, is a simple answer. He refers us to a paper published in 1956, by George A. Miller, called 'The Magical Number 7 Plus or Minus 2: Some Limits on Our Capacity for Processing Information'. In the article, which has become a classic, and has been cited in no fewer than 4,500 academic papers since it was written, Miller suggests that, in a number of areas, the human mind seems to have limits to the amount of information that can be processed at a time, and in particular that about seven items of information is that limit.

First of all, let me give a very simple example of how that might work. In 2007 *The Times* published a puzzle in its Daily Workout section similar to the following:

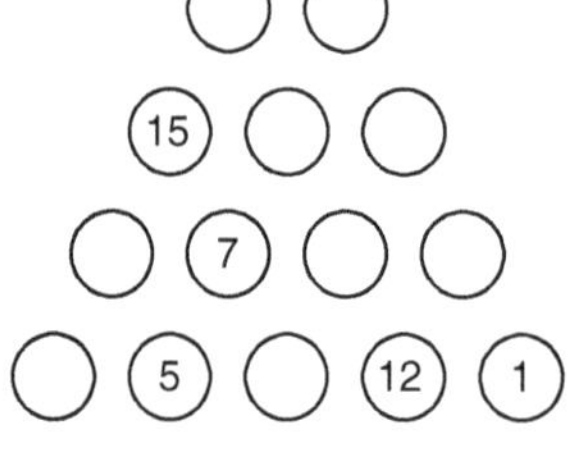

'Add Up: The number in each circle is the sum of the two below it. Work out the top number. Try it in your head, if you can'.

15 = 7 + 8, so the number in the first circle in the second row must be 8. Similarly, 7 = 5 + 2, so the middle number on the bottom row must be 2. If we put those numbers into the puzzle pyramid, the result is:

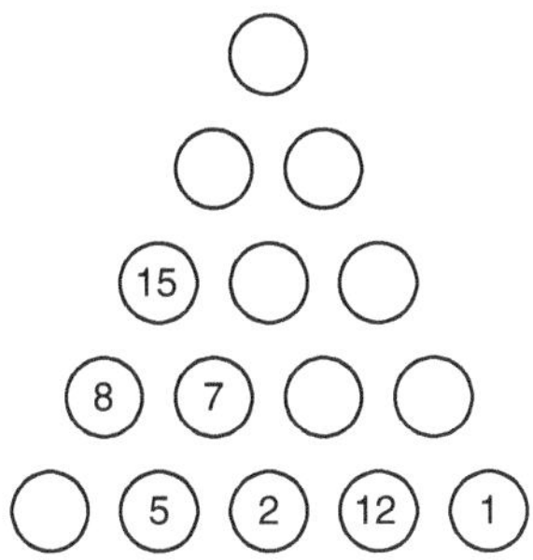

Similar reasoning gives the answer that the remaining number on the bottom line is 3, although calculating it is not strictly necessary.

After that we can work our way up the pyramid by simply adding the numbers together. A next step might be:

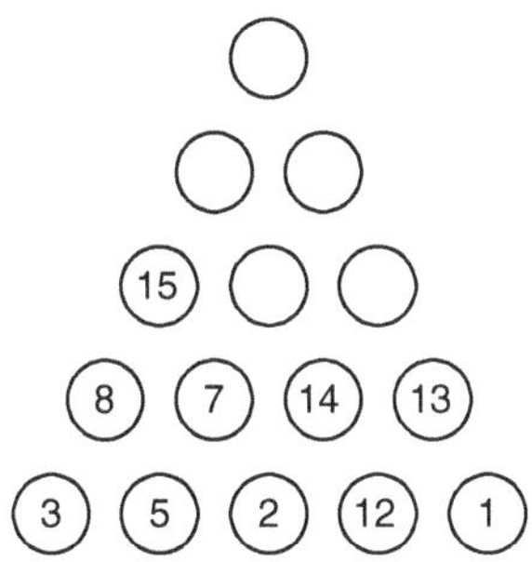

The pyramid can then be relatively simply completed:

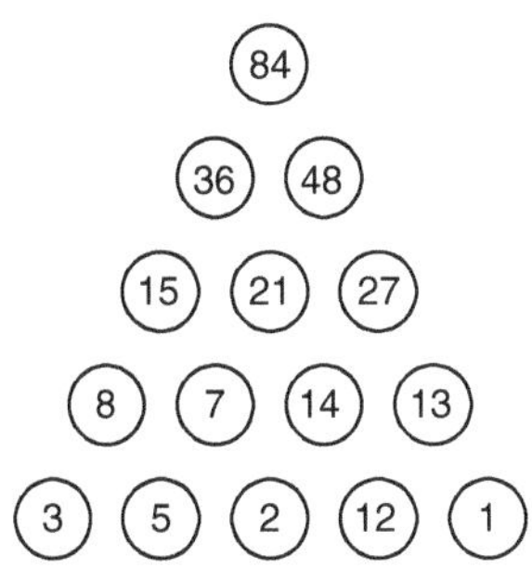

The most difficult mental arithmetic operation that is required is 36 + 48 = 84. In those terms, it is not very difficult. However, if we add in the injunction to try to work it out in our head, without writing down any of the intermediate answers, the task becomes very much more difficult. At the same time as performing all those little addition sums, one has to remember the numbers that are to be entered into the circles in the pyramid. There are 10 blank circles in the original puzzle, so that in order to find the answer we will probably need to keep in mind 10 numbers at the same time as performing the last addition. Interestingly, this exceeds Miller's magical number seven, and it is by no means easy to do – you may wish to try.

Lynch takes this as a starting point, or perhaps better a metaphor, in order to explain what it would be like to think beyond the range of normal human beings. He speculates that, since the majority of us are stuck with a limit of about seven items in active memory, genius may consist in being able to juggle a dozen, or even a score of items in active memory. As a simple metaphor this has some attractions. More memory equals better thinking. I certainly know that if I plug an extra gigabyte or two into the motherboard of my computer it will be able to run programs more efficiently than it does now, and may even be able to run some programs that are beyond its capacity now. And it plays into the idea of smart drugs, and the physical basis for intellectual ability, rather well. If thinking and memory are processes which depend upon the creation of connections between neighbouring neurons, then more connections may equate with better thinking. If we can increase the flow of oxygen to those brain cells, or in some other way make it possible for them to connect in more complex ways, new thoughts may be possible.

The first thing to note is that Miller did not say what Lynch reports him as saying. Lynch argues that there is a limit to the amount of information that the human brain can handle, and that this limit can only be overcome by the physical improvement of the brain. Miller is much more careful in his conclusions than that, and actually points to ways in which people can learn to handle more information without an improvement in their brain. Lynch describes Miller's conclusions in a way that seems to support Lynch's arguments, and which does serious damage to the care with which Miller actually expressed himself. One has to be very charitable indeed to suppose that this misinterpretation of Miller is accidental rather than a wilful misinterpretation of Miller's findings. Miller most decidedly not conclude that his findings imply a limit to how well we can think, or that new ideas must wait upon the improvement of the brain. Perhaps it would be best to start by examining what Miller actually said.

First he presented reports on a number of research projects relating to mental capacity. These included laboratory experiments involving subjects distinguishing between different stimuli, such as the pitch of notes or the positioning of pointers, as well as more conventional tests of active memory, where subjects are asked to remember lists of digits or nonsense syllables. In all cases, there appeared to be some kind of limit, around the number seven, to the mental capacity of those tested. It seems that subjects can typically distinguish up to six different notes, but not more, for example. And this limit appears to be independent of how those stimuli are arranged, for example how widely they are spread over a frequency range.

This seems paradoxical. As Miller notes:

> For example, if you can discriminate five high-pitched tones in one series and five low-pitched tones in another series, it is reasonable to expect that you could combine all ten into a single series and still tell them apart without error. When you try it, however, it does not work. The channel capacity for pitch seems to be about six and that is the best that you can do.

This reference to 'channel capacity' is taken from the explanation that Miller constructs about the amount of information that is transmitted by a signal, such as a note of a particular pitch. Miller is arguing, at least in part, that the limit to a person's capacity to distinguish stimuli and remember digits can best be described as a limit to the amount of information that he or she can process. Miller stops short of suggesting that there is a common mechanism that underlies the appearance of this limit in different areas of mental activity, a caution that Lynch might have done well to emulate.

The second half of the paper addresses this question of whether a person faces an absolute limit as to the amount of information that they can process at a particular time. For example, a numerical digit conveys less information than a letter of the alphabet; a digit would allow one to correctly identify a member of a class of 10, while a letter would allow one to identify a member of a class of 26. Consequently, if the human brain suffered from an absolute limit to the amount of information that it could process at a particular time, a person should be able to remember a shorter string of random letters than of random numerical digits. It should be easier to remember 451973 than to remember DKLWXB, because there are a million 6-digit numbers to choose from, and over three hundred million combinations that can be made up from 6 letters. That is to say, the string of 6 letters can convey three hundred times the amount of information that can be conveyed by the 6-digit number. But this is not at all what happens. It appears that the two sequences are more or less equally easy to remember. And certainly, the 6 letters are not three hundred times as difficult to remember.

Miller accounts for this by describing a process which he calls 'chunking' or 'recoding'. A person can reorganize information into familiar groupings or chunks which make the information easier to remember. In an experiment conducted by Smith, experts familiar with different number systems were asked to remember strings of binary digits, by reorganizing them into numbers in base 8, base 16 and base 32. As a consequence of collecting the same information together into larger chunks, it was easier for the subjects to retain the information. It is this process of chunking that is of interest to Miller, rather than the absolute limit that seems to be represented by the remembering of seven chunks.

To put this another way, the specialist in a field and the novice may each recall seven things about that field of study. But the expert's seven items will be complex chunks that they can use to recall a range of sub-chunks of information. The expert has developed a classification system and a range of techniques with which he or she is familiar, and which make it possible to manipulate much larger quantities of information. As Miller puts it: '[T]he process of recoding is a very important one in human psychology and deserves much more explicit attention than it has received. In particular, the kind of linguistic recoding that people do seems to me to be the very lifeblood of the thought processes . . . yet, probably because recoding is less accessible to experimental manipulation than nonsense syllables or T mazes, the traditional experimental psychologist has contributed little or nothing to their analysis'.

I find this reminiscent of Vygotsky's observation that, because psychologists try to examine everything in terms of stimulus–response, psychology is much more successful at accounting for lower mental functions than for higher mental functions. And although Miller's commentary was written in the mid-1950s, it stands as an appropriate rebuke to Lynch who seeks to use this paper to suggest a limit to normal thought which can be overcome by the use of pharmaceuticals. In fact, Miller's paper is primarily about techniques which people use routinely to overcome that 'limit'. Recoding is the most important, but the paper also touches upon others, such as organizing stimuli on several different dimensions.

To reiterate, people regularly overcome the problem of handling more information by using techniques to organize the task before them differently. Let me illustrate this by returning once again to the number pyramid, but this time offer a technique which will dramatically reduce the amount of memory required. Consider the bottom row of the pyramid alone:

(3) (5) (2) (12) (1)

Now it happens that the top number in the pyramid can be calculated by adding the outside two numbers to four times the next two numbers in and six times the central number, or adding 3, 20, 12, 48 and 1.* The rest of the pyramid is irrelevant. So long as a person is

* If the numbers in the bottom line are a, b, c, d and e, then the numbers in the next line up are $(a + b)$, $(b + c)$, $(c + d)$ and $(d + e)$.

Similarly, the three numbers in the next line are:

$(a + b + b + c)$, $(b + c + c + d)$ and $(c + d + d + e)$,
i.e. $(a + 2b + c)$, $(b + 2c + d)$ and $(c + 2d + e)$.

The two numbers in the penultimate line are:

$(a + 2b + c + b + 2c + d)$ and $(b + 2c + d + c + 2d + e)$,
i.e. $(a + 3b + 3c + d)$ and $(b + 3c + 3d + e)$.

That means that the top number is $(a + 3b + 3c + d + b + 3c + 3d + e)$,
i.e. $(a + 4b + 6c + 4d + e)$.

very familiar with their four and six times table (so that multiplying by four or six does not occupy a lot of mental process), he or she can calculate the top number of the pyramid while remembering only 5 digits, 3 of which were printed in the original puzzle. This dramatically reduces the processing load, while always giving the correct answer.

This means that we have to re-examine Lynch's suggestion that we might imagine what it is like to be a genius, or be able to imagine how our thinking might be enhanced by taking smart drugs, by thinking that it could enable us to hold more information in active memory than was otherwise the case. This is not only not what Miller said, but it is necessary to wilfully misinterpret Miller in order to arrive at Lynch's conclusion. Miller said that people routinely exceed their own capacity, and they routinely exceed it by learning, internalizing and becoming very familiar with coding frames which allow them to recode the information that they are thinking about. Such coding frames include the alphabet, counting systems, multiplication tables and many others, each of which is a socially constructed way of organizing thought in a helpful way. Vygotsky also spoke of how learning involves the incorporation of such classificatory frameworks into our 'natural' thought processes in order to enhance, or develop, our higher mental functions. He gave the example of memory, where certain processes, which he described as techno-mnemonic could be added to our unaided, or mnemonic, memory. However, in the course of time, those techno-mnemonic processes become internalized as part of our 'natural' or automatic thought processes, and with increasing familiarity become indistinguishable from the original capacity of the brain. We see here a process through which learning enhances the mental capacity and allows us to transcend any boundary which may appear to present itself.

In order to illustrate this more fully, it would perhaps be sensible to look at another interpretation of Miller's work which is more faithful to the original intent. This is the theory of cognitive load, developed by Paul Ayres and John Sweller.

The idea of cognitive load theory is that, at any given point in time, there will be a limit to the amount of information that a person can process. Thus, if we wish a person to learn something, there is absolutely no point in trying to teach them at the same time as loading them up with unnecessary memory requirements. For example, a person who is using the pyramid puzzle as a means of practising simple arithmetic will be completely overloaded if we ask them to work it out in their head (as I expect the demonstration has already shown). In order to teach a person we need to make sure that we frame the essential tasks so that they fall within the person's current capacity.

As a slight aside, there may be a range of hints in Miller's paper as to how this might be done. Miller reported results that showed that arranging judgements along several dimensions (such as colour, shape and size, for example) would increase the ability to distinguish between stimuli (shapes projected onto a screen) – for example an ability to distinguish quickly between three different shapes of three different colours would be easier than distinguishing nine different shapes or nine different colours. However, while different dimensions added to the range of stimuli that could be distinguished, the process was not strictly additive. More stimuli could be distinguished, but not quite as many as would be expected by simply adding together the capabilities on each of the stimuli separately.

This hint is full of possibilities for how multimedia stimuli might be used to reduce the cognitive load on the learner when presenting information. The outcome is not quite as clear as one might initially suppose, however, if one assumes that using more media necessarily increases the range of material that a person can handle. It seems that integrating material from information from different media, say visual and auditory, is a cognitive task in its own right, and that, consequently, gratuitous use of multimedia can in fact increase cognitive load and make it more difficult to take in information.

The other aspect of Miller's work that is relevant to learning, however, is recoding. If the material presented is too comfortably within the capacity of the learner, he or she will have little incentive to recode, or, which is the same thing, to develop new mental classifications and frameworks. The task should therefore be within the learner's capacity, but not too far within the capacity that there is no stimulus to reorganize his or her ways of thinking. Bearing in mind that it will take some mental capacity to learn, presenting tasks which fully occupy the learner's mental capacity, or exceed it, will make teaching completely fruitless.

Thus, in discussing cognitive load theory, van Merriënboer and Ayres (2005) note three kinds of cognitive load: (a) intrinsic cognitive load, (b) extraneous cognitive load and (c) germane cognitive load.

(a) Intrinsic cognitive load is the mental capacity that needs to be devoted to the specific task. It is important to note, however, that the description offered by van Merriënboer and Ayres does not suggest that this is fixed for a specific task irrespective of the person doing the task and their prior experience. An expert in a field will have at his or her disposal techniques, and most particularly mental schema, which allow them to tackle more complex tasks with less mental effort, or making fewer demands on active memory.
(b) Extraneous cognitive load is the cognitive load which arises because of the process of instruction, and is not necessary for the learning process. We might think, for example, of complex language used by the teacher, which impose an additional burden of 'translation' upon the novice in order to come to grips with the substance of the lesson. In most cases it will be desirable to reduce the extraneous cognitive load through careful instructional design. (I say 'in most cases' because it is quite possible to imagine cases where high levels of extraneous cognitive load would be desirable; when training experts to screen out irrelevant stimuli, for example, learning to cope with extraneous cognitive load may be the point and purpose of the exercise.) What cognitive load theory suggests is that it is extremely important for teachers and instructors to understand the management of extraneous cognitive load.
(c) Germane cognitive load is the cognitive load which is directly associated with the process of learning, for example where a process of adopting a new schema or reinterpreting previously held knowledge in the light of that new schema is required. Again, it should be noted that van Merriënboer and Ayres do not suggest that there is anything mechanical about this. Simply because a person is not overloaded in terms of intrinsic cognitive load or extraneous cognitive load, does not mean that they will devote their available mental capacity to learning. They also have to be

motivated to apply themselves to learning, and see the practical importance of that learning in their own situation.

van Merriënboer and Ayres give a useful table (Table 1) summarizing the main effects that have been studied using cognitive load theory.

Table 1 Traditional effects studied by CLT and why they reduce extraneous cognitive load (reported by Sweller, van Merriënboer and Paas, 1998)

Effect	Description	Extraneous Load
Goal-Free effect	Replace conventional problems with goal-free problems, which provide learners with a non-specific goal	Reduces extraneous cognitive load caused by relating a current problem state to a goal state and attempting to reduce differences between them; focuses learner's attention on problem states and available operators
Worked Example effect	Replace conventional problems with worked examples that must be carefully studied	Reduces extraneous cognitive load caused by weak-method problem solving; focuses learner's attention on problem states and useful solution steps
Completion Problem effect	Replace conventional problems with completion problems, provides a partial solution that must be completed by the learners	Reduces extraneous cognitive load because giving part of the solution reduces the size of the problem space; focuses attention on problem states and useful solution steps
Split Attention effect	Replace multiple sources of information (frequently pictures and accompanying text) with a single, integrated source of information	Reduces extraneous cognitive load because there is no need to mentally integrate the information sources
Modality effect	Replace a written explanatory text and another source of visual information such as a diagram (unimodal) with a spoken explanatory text and a visual source of information (multimodal)	Reduces extraneous cognitive load because the multimodal presentation uses both the visual and auditory processor of working memory
Redundancy effect	Replace multiple sources of information that are self-contained (i.e., they can be understood on their own) with one source of information	Reduces extraneous cognitive load caused by unnecessary processing of redundant information

Source: With kind permission from Springer Science+Business Media: John Sweller, 1998 'Cognitive Architecture and Instructional Design' in *Educational Psychology Review*, Vol. 10, pp. 251–296.

Chapter 6

Attention Deficit

In May 2008 the Academy of Medical Sciences (2008) published a report by a working group on *Brain Science, Addiction and Drugs*, a major part of which was devoted to the use of cognition enhancing drugs, or 'smart drugs'. While this was, in many ways, an attempt to present a balanced discussion of the issues around the use of cognition enhancing drugs, it was, in fact, seriously biased in two important respects. First, it was very firmly based upon a medical model of intelligence, and the idea that knowledge and memory depend essentially upon the physical mechanism that is used to express them. And secondly, and perhaps as a direct consequence of that, it slipped rather too often into the assumption that cognition enhancing drugs, in some form or another, work.

In this chapter I will use that report as a measure of how the medical model of brain function shapes our thinking about learning. And against that background, I will develop an alternative, constructivist view of intelligence and learning, derived from the theories of Vygotsky and Mead, which presents learning as social, language and culture as mechanisms for self-control, and meta-cognition, knowledge about what is known, as being as important as or more important than the actual content of what is known. It will look at learning as the development of the ability to focus one's own attention.

In effect, we have two very different ways of thinking about the functioning of the brain and mind. In one, forgetting is seen as something pathological, a malfunction of the person, which needs to be treated and corrected. In the other, forgetting is a normal function of life, which we all experience to a greater or lesser extent, but which we can manage by employing a variety of techniques judiciously. It may even be the case, if we think for a moment about how overwhelmed we would be if we never forgot anything, that forgetting has a positive function in helping us to cope with unpleasant experiences, or to select the most relevant information.

Much the same applies to the ability to focus one's attention, which in the medical model should be enhanced if deficient through the use of drugs such as ritalin. On the constructivist view, managing one's attention is something that each of us has to learn how to do, and at which one can become better over time with experience. However, that tendency that we all have to find our minds wandering from the subject in hand may also be a benefit, as when one is taken from reading a book by a beautiful sunset, or perhaps notices a happy conjunction of idea that leads to a serendipitous discovery.

In the former view we are born with certain capabilities, and if we are not as good as the next person at remembering, or focusing our attention, then we are exhibiting symptoms of a syndrome that should be treated. On the latter view we are simply experiencing part of that wide diversity which is part of the human condition.

One of the opening paragraphs of Academy of Medical Sciences' report explained why there is currently such a high level of interest in cognition enhancing drugs:

> Much of the recent attention directed towards cognition enhancers is due to the pharmaceutical industry's interest in treatments for dementia (including Alzheimer's disease, Pick's disease and Lewy body dementia, as well as the dementia associated with Parkinson's disease) and, more recently, stroke, schizophrenia and Attention Deficit Hyperactivity Disorder (ADHD). The economic arguments underpinning this interest are compelling, given the prevalence of these disorders and the potential market for effective therapies. (Academy of Medical Sciences, 2008: 146)

This is interesting for a number of reasons, both in stressing the medical basis for the interest in such drugs, but also in stressing the very large economic interests that are involved. However, this comment should, perhaps, be taken together with a reflection from the discussion of cognition enhancing drugs, where the report stated, 'The Foresight project concluded that pharmaceutical companies have not pursued cognition enhancing drugs for use in the healthy population because of perceived regulation and litigation issues that enhance commercial risk' (Academy of Medical Sciences, 2008: 158).

There is a line of reasoning here, which suggests that pharmaceutical companies are not pursuing (and perhaps should not pursue) the development of drugs which enhance the cognition of normal, healthy people. But this is linked to the idea that ADHD, which at the very best is a rather loose collection of symptoms, is to be classified as a disease, and is therefore suitable for treatment (and, by implication, economic exploitation).

It is worth taking a brief diversion here into Vygotsky's theory of learning. Vygotsky suggested that we are born with certain native reflexes, such as turning our attention to loud noises. We can, however, be taught to focus our attention on other stimuli – our mother's voice, somebody calling our name, and by degrees ever more finely graduated symbols that can be used to guide attention. Eventually, having seen not only how others can manage our attention using language, but also how we can manage the attention of others in a similar way, we come to an understanding of how we can manage our own attention using symbols. I promise myself a break and a cup of coffee after working on this book for half an hour, or I manage my environment to reduce the likelihood of distractions that I do not wish to pay attention to.

'Attention deficit' is a very interesting concept. It is, after all, highly context specific. If I am cornered at a cocktail party by somebody who wishes to talk about fly fishing or motor racing, or something else that I have no interest in, I am likely to find my concentration wandering, as I speculate whether there is somebody more interesting in the room that I might talk to. I might even feel moved to get up and walk away. But if the conversation was engrossing me, I would have relatively little difficulty concentrating on the details. I would hardly think that I had contracted a disease at the party by coming into contact with people who might be contagious. On the other hand, if I only ever came into contact with people who talked about matters that were of no interest to me, and for which I could see no practical purpose, then I might well not develop those habits of critical and active listening which, through careful practice, I have now developed so that I can use them at will.

The idea that self-management of our attention is something that we are born with, and that if a child is distracted this means they are suffering form a medical condition, is really very extraordinary. Children show very great powers of concentration on matters that interest them, and through practice can also employ them on matters that are of less interest to them. All of our higher mental abilities are developed over time with practice, and the ability to listen courteously to something that is of little interest is something that we take on board as part of our adult responsibilities. Children are different from adults, in a variety of ways – the proportions of their bodies, the development of their bones and muscles, their ability to sit still and concentrate for long periods on dull matter – but, with the exception of the last, these are not generally seen as disorders. Of course there are extreme cases, but most of us fall within a range that, as we grow, means that we develop out of those conditions.

It will be important to return to the question of what is, or is not, natural in the way that we think. The conclusion that we need to take away from Vygotsky's work is that there are very few adults who think in a way that is 'natural'. We have incorporated into the way that we think techniques and symbols that we have drawn from the culture in which we were raised so that we can think in better ways. Do I think in the same way as a person from the stone age, or even from the fourteenth century? Absolutely, I do not. A person from the stone age, or from the fourteenth century, could not use differential calculus. He or she had a different notion of perspective than I do. And he or she knew nothing of modern technology, and could therefore not compare the action of the heart with that of a pump, or that of the brain with the action of a computer. (Whether such metaphors help or hinder my thinking is not the point here; those metaphors, for better or worse, were not available to people from earlier centuries.) There is nothing 'natural' about the way that we think. Our thinking is enhanced, but it is enhanced by the incorporation of ways of thinking, of conceptual frameworks, of thinking schema and so on.

In contrast with that, do I have a brain that is similar to that of a person from the stone age or the fourteenth century? Yes, I do. Very little in brain physiology has changed in centuries, and that raises important questions about the too ready reliance on the idea that thought, memory and intelligence have a directly physical basis. The most important parts of human thought, that is to say those parts that are most characteristically human, do not leave a physical trace in the brain.

This means that it is very important to weigh carefully what it is that we need to believe if we are to suppose that there may be cognition enhancing drugs, and what, in this report, is being taken for granted. First, the pharmaceutical companies are addressing what seems to me to be a primitive need for reassurance in most people that they are not interfering in the 'natural'. Drugs are being developed to cure diseases. But that also means that if there is a widely prevalent condition that they think they can provide drugs for, they must manage to convince us that it is pathological, as is the case with ADHD. In spite of the fact that we send children to school for 12 years or more in an effort to induce them to adopt unnatural ways of thinking, the report specifically notes the attachment that the general public seems to have to supposedly natural ways of conducting oneself, and the paradoxes that this leads to: 'For instance, it was seen as much more desirable to add cognition enhancers to food such as broccoli; the idea of feeding "enhanced broccoli" to one's family was viewed far more favourably than dosing a child with a pill before going to school' (Academy of Medical Sciences, 2008: 149).

This fluidity about whether what we are looking at are illnesses or not can be moved decisively in favour of the pharmaceutical companies by suggesting that all of us experience pathological failures of cognition from time to time, and of course, the more often we experience them, the more legitimate will the routine use of cognition enhancing drugs become. 'How is it possible to boost cognitive function in healthy individuals, if they already perform at or near the optimum? The reason is that normal cognition often strays from optimum, for example as a function of fatigue, sleep deprivation or stress' (Academy of Medical Sciences, 2008: 153). That is to say, we all know that we under-perform on occasions, and that, consequently, we might bring ourselves back to peak performance with the use of cognition enhancing drugs.

It is curious, since the report refers to the comparison with the use of performance enhancing drugs in sport which is often used, that the analogy should not be followed to its logical conclusion. Would it be acceptable for sportsmen and women to use drugs on the days when their performance was a little below par? In most drug testing regimes, it would not; the use of drugs to enhance performance is absolutely prohibited.

However, this model of cognition enhancing drugs, as bringing us back up to some supposedly natural, optimal level of performance, leads to further confusions and complications. Although we actually know very little about how a specific mental process would be given expression in the brain, it is generally assumed (perhaps it is the only sensible assumption and quite possibly correct) that thoughts are propagated by chains of neurons, each one passing a message to others that are interconnected with it. For this to be a feasible mechanism, however, the brain cannot be constructed entirely of neurons which excite other interconnected neurons. Such a brain would be subject to ever-increasing bouts of excitation which never ended. The brain must also incorporate mechanisms for damping down cell activity, neurons that inhibit the action of other cells once the thought has passed. The brain must be a careful balance of excitation and inhibition so that thoughts, our important thoughts, can develop but not be drowned out by a multitude of other, secondary signals.

If we wish to enhance cognitive function, do we need more excitation, or do we need more inhibition? Or, perhaps, do we already have exactly the right amount of both, and any disturbance of that balance might actually impair our cognitive functions? The report suggests that the latter might be the case, by arguing that the relationship between neurotransmitter function and cognitive function is in the shape of an inverted U (Academy of Medical Sciences, 2008: 150). That is to say, there is an optimal balance and that moving either way will upset cognitive function. The report notes a number of consequences of this, not least that different levels of excitation may be appropriate for different cognitive functions. In addition, it implies that drugs will act differently in 'normal' subjects than in those who have some permanent imbalance in their neurochemistry. All of this points to the need for extreme caution when interpreting the results of tests with cognition enhancing drugs. I do not think that the need for caution would be disputed, and the report highlights this on several occasions. It remains an open question, however, whether the report exemplifies an appropriate level of caution.

We should not then be surprised that the report includes this description of cognition enhancing drugs: 'Research has shown that most of the pharmaceutical drugs act to enhance (or diminish) neurotransmitter function and synaptic efficacy' (Academy of Medical Sciences, 2008: 143). That rather interesting admission that we are not sure whether we ought to be trying to enhance or diminish neurotransmitter function should at least give us a hint as to the true state of medical knowledge in this field. Those with knowledge of the medical sciences are generally keen to stress, as this report does, that we know relatively little at the moment, and that useful applications are a long way off, but they invariably follow that with the very great promise that research in this field holds out, and, of course, that more research is necessary. Medical solutions appear to hold such promise.

'However, small percentage increments in performance can lead to significant improvements in functional outcome; it is conceivable that a 10% improvement in memory score could lead to an improvement in an A-level grade or degree class' (Academy of Medical Sciences, 2008: 150). If such a modest improvement in performance could turn mediocre students into excellent students, this seems to be a prize well worth investing in. This should give us pause for thought, but not, I hope, in a medical line of argument. If memory alone can account for a grade or two or a degree class or two, could we not design tests that are able to measure more important mental capacities, since we will rarely ask graduates to perform a task on the basis of their memory, but will expect them to make full use of reference libraries and information sources in forming their judgements. But this does lead us rather importantly to the question of what kind of tests are being used to measure cognitive enhancement. What, exactly, counts as cognitive enhancement, and how close is it to anything that we might think was valuable in everyday life?

The report puts this question in a rather similar form, and appears to suggest an answer:

> Researchers will need to explore novel approaches to evaluating the effects of cognition enhancers in healthy individuals, particularly

> in relating laboratory evaluations to everyday functional outcomes. For instance, how does the laboratory observation that modafinil enables human volunteers to hold an average of seven digits in short term memory, rather than six, relate to everyday performance, say in planning a shopping trip or in enhancing performance in the workplace? To validate laboratory measures as predictors of real life effects, researchers will have to be able to measure such everyday performance in significantly better ways than at present. (Academy of Medical Sciences, 2008: 158)

That is to say, after taking a dose of modafinil, human volunteers were able to hold an average of seven digits in short term memory rather than six. Before dismissing such evidence as nonsense, it is perhaps worth considering why it is important that the tests were conducted on such very low level activities. In the previous chapter I referred to work derived from the insights provided by Miller that showed that what we can keep in our memories is critically linked to how we chunk information, and what techniques, classifications and schema we are familiar with for managing memory. If cognition enhancing drugs were tested in circumstances where chunking effects and the effects of prior knowledge might influence the outcome, any possible effects of the drugs would be swamped by the things that are actually important in human memory. In order to see the effects of drugs at all it is necessary that the tests be conducted on tasks that are extremely simple. So simple, in fact, as to rule out the influence of higher mental functions at all.

Suppose, for example, that we take a simple technique for remembering random digits, which many people use for remembering PIN numbers, namely visualizing a sequence of key strokes on a telephone key pad. This might make it possible for a person to memorize an additional digit, say seven digits instead of six. There are many such methods for remembering sequences of random digits. Breaking them down into dates is a common one. My personal favourite is to group numbers into the numbers of bus routes that have played an important part in my life. Other people will have other methods. Each of these mnemono-technical methods can have an impact on performance in memory tests comparable to the size of the effect of drugs, and that effect will increase as the task becomes more complex. Therefore any test of the efficacy of drugs is likely to interfere with the results obtained. Some people may be using mnemonotechnical methods and others may not, while a few may even adopt them during the tests.

In case it should be thought that I am trying to criticize the testing procedures used to test cognition enhancing drugs by selecting the most trivial of tests, I should stress that I am not. If I wanted to do that, I might point to the drug tests where apes are trained to respond to shapes that are projected on the screen of a computer, and then tested for their reactions after they have been deprived of sleep (Lynch, 2006). And the issue here is not that sleep deprived chimpanzees are as far removed as one can hope to get from everyday human experience. The point is that when testing chimpanzees the mental associations of the stars and circles and crescents displayed on the screen can be ignored. The idea that the chimpanzee might be especially motivated, for some reason, to struggle against tiredness can be ignored. In fact, anything human in terms of thought processes can be eliminated so that the action of the cognition enhancing drugs can be studied.

But even more interestingly, the report does not conclude that it would be foolish to infer anything from drug tests and transfer it to more complex human activities. On the contrary, it suggests that, 'researchers will have to be able to measure such everyday performance in significantly better ways than at present'. The only thing that can possibly mean is that everyday performance will have to be broken down into insignificant pieces that fit into the kind of double blind drug trials that medicine demands. Do not let us suppose for one minute that teachers or educationists may have some insight into how everyday performance might be measured and evaluated. Let us hand that task over to medical researchers. Perhaps we already have, in our endless search for basic, transferable skills and testable competencies. Cognition enhancing drugs may have no discernible benefit for the normal, healthy learner, but the idea of them may already be having a terrible, deleterious effect on the education of millions.

Currently the main candidate as cognition enhancing drug of choice, which is readily available on the internet, is modafinil.

On the specific subject of modafinil, the report had the following to say:

> Modafinil (Provigil) is licensed in the UK for treating the excessive daytime sleepiness associated with narcolepsy and disorders of breathing during sleep (sleep apnoea). The drug is also used in the treatment of sleep disorders resulting from shift-work. Recent studies have shown that non-sleep deprived volunteers may also benefit in certain domains of cognitive function. For instance, tests in young adults have shown improvements in verbal working memory, visual recognition, planning performance and executive inhibitory control (stop-signal reaction time) (Randall et al., 2003; Turner et al., 2003b [Turner et al., 2003]; Muller et al., 2004). However, improvements were not seen in other tests of learning and memory, suggesting that the beneficial effects of modafinil may be limited to particular brain systems. Clinical trials and laboratory studies of modafinil have shown improvements in cognitive function in cases of ADHD (Turner et al., 2004a) and schizophrenia (Turner et al., 2004b). However, in the USA, the licensing for the use of modafinil to treat ADHD has been delayed by reports of rare dermatological side effects. The beneficial effects of modafinil, and its lack of obvious toxic effects or apparent abuse liability (Myrick et al., 2004), appear to have led to considerable 'offlabel' use of this compound, in addition to its recent use by the USA military. (Academy of Medical Sciences, 2008: 150–1)

I have quoted this at length because I think that it is important to acknowledge that these drugs may have some beneficial effects. While I have some doubts about ADHD, as noted above, I have no wish to suggest that we should not be looking for drugs which help in the treatment of schizophrenia. But even if one is trying to be a even handed as possible, it is difficult to avoid the fact that this paragraph presents a rather confused picture, of a drug that lacks 'obvious toxic effects' but has failed to satisfy the licensing authorities in the USA because of its side effects (the less serious of which are not even mentioned).

And there seems to be still more confusion in the idea of a drug that lacks 'apparent abuse liability' at the same time as exhibiting 'considerable "offlabel" use', elsewhere estimated at $500 million a year. In so much confusion, one thing appears absolutely clear; a general faith among the authors of the report and the members of the public that they engaged in their enquiries that such drugs could bring about cognitive enhancement.

When listing the concerns that the general public harboured in relation to the widespread use of cognition enhancing drugs, the report had this to say:

> **Public engagement: concerns**
>
> It is clear from the results of the public engagement programme that most of the hopes for cognition enhancers focus on their potential use in helping people who are ill, rather than enhancing the 'well'. Participants cited several concerns related to the possibility of cognition enhancers becoming widely available for use by healthy adults. These can be broadly categorised as follows:
>
> 1. Unwanted or unknown side effects, related to a general fear of addiction and the absence of information about their long term effects.
> 2. Devaluation of 'normal' achievements and the potential reduction in the intrinsic value of the effort and motivation involved in learning.
> 3. Inequality, particularly if such drugs were expensive.
> 4. Pressure to use and exacerbation of an already over-competitive culture.
> 5. Control of people's behaviour.
> 6. Personality change, perhaps resulting from long-term use. (Academy of Medical Sciences, 2008: 156)

It is noticeable that all of the concerns which were central to the public resulted from a belief that the drugs work. It is not possible to be concerned that the use of drugs might devalue 'normal' achievement, or bring about a drug divide in society, or lead to increased competitiveness, unless one first believes that the drugs actually do have the desired effect of enhancing cognitive performance, and that in areas that have a significant impact in everyday life. Even the other concerns are concerns about side effects, and there would be little need to worry about the side effects or long term use if the drugs did not have some effects that were seen as primary and beneficial. Why is it that we find it so easy to imagine that such drugs could work?

Before leaving this question, it would perhaps be appropriate to note that the balanced views expressed in the report of the Academy of Medical Sciences are by no means the only ones to be found in the public arena. The *New Scientist* of 13 December 2008 carried a story under the headline 'Go brain-boosters'. The report, which was based on an article in *Nature*, summarized the gist of the report: 'Society should embrace the use of drugs that boost brain power. That's the message from a group of neuroscientists, psychiatrists and ethicists' ('Go Brain-boosters', 2008).

The report in the *New Scientist* concludes with a comment from Julian Savulescu: 'Brain pills could give an edge to nations whose citizens opt to raise their intelligence, suggests neuroethicist Julian Savulescu of the University of Oxford'. Although this comment does not come from one of the many co-authors of the *Nature* paper, it is clearly designed to bolster the idea that cognition enhancement is ethically unobjectionable. However, the case is somewhat weakened by the fact that Savulescu, in spite of being a 'neuroethicist', seems to be able to embrace almost any use of drugs for performance enhancement, in all spheres of activity. As another newspaper report makes clear, 'It [sport] is another one of the realms in which he has attracted controversy – unlike many people, he has no moral problem with sportspeople using performance enhancing drugs. "The whole concept that performance-enhancement itself is against the spirit of sport is wrong" he says' (Maley, 2008).

Returning to the original report in *Nature*, however, it is clear that the 'commentary' is far from neutral. Cognition enhancement is presented as being the moral equivalent of drinking coffee, and improving human beings is argued to be a moral obligation, rather than an activity that needs to be weighed carefully.

> Many people have doubts about the moral status of enhancement drugs for reasons ranging from the pragmatic to the philosophical, including concerns about short-circuiting personal agency and

or adornments to their role as citizens, such as the application of their professional perspective to political and social questions, but we do very little to address those areas explicitly. As somebody who is committed to higher education, I am persuaded that studying for a degree does produce an approach to difficult issues and a confidence to tackle them which is invaluable. I value the qualities of graduates who leave university after several years of conscientious study. But in saying that, it is rarely the quality of the specialist knowledge which prepares them to take up a professional role in society.

This is not a phenomenon that is restricted to higher education. Secondary school curricula are designed primarily to prepare young people for their study in higher education. Those who leave formal education at the end of secondary schooling have, for the most part, a preparation for a course of action that they do not intend to pursue. Similarly primary school is largely shaped in the image of what is needed in order to be successful in secondary school, and we are now looking at ways of making pre-school an appropriate preparation for primary school. (This was not always the case; in the pre-Plowden years, primary schools were freer from this pressure to prepare children with the skills that were needed in secondary schools. The National Curriculum, key stages of development and standard attainment targets have driven primary schools to see themselves as preparation for secondary school. And we are in the process of seeing this extended further to kindergartens, reception classes and childminders.)

And this is not a criticism that can be answered by pointing to 'vocational' courses in schools and colleges. Those vocational courses are, for the most part, shaped by the expectations of teachers who have been brought up in an academic tradition, and who are trying to 'cope' with students who are not adequately prepared or motivated to follow the academic curriculum. The result is a nasty hybrid of what a subject specialist thinks would be appropriate for somebody who is not smart enough to follow the proper course of study.

The real problem lies elsewhere. We are in the process of changing our society so as to remove the possible occupations of whole swathes of the population. To understand what this means you would need to go to a plumbers' merchant or builders' merchant at 8 o'clock on a weekday morning. The store will be full of people who have immense expertise. They may possibly be holding dirty scraps of paper with shopping lists written on them. If they do, those shopping lists will probably be appallingly misspelt, to the extent that you, who are used to reading standard spelling of the type that you find in this book, would have difficulty deciphering them. Explain to the group of people what you are attempting to do, and why you are there to buy parts, and you will find a wealth of expertise, from how to wipe a joint in a lead pipe to how to replace a stretch of guttering, because this early morning meeting is, in part, a social and learning event. It is the seminar of a community of practice.

These skilled men and women are the repository of a huge range of experience and skills. For the most part we would describe them as functionally illiterate. That is to say, of course, that they would fail a test set by an academic. In practice, their literacy is perfectly matched to their required functions of writing shopping lists that they can understand but nobody else needs to. But their skills are being progressively phased out of our society. Nobody wipes a soldered joint these days, not only because people prefer not to drink water that has been supplied through lead pipes, but also because it is difficult to do and requires skill. Instead, we manufacture plastic piping that requires less skill to assemble. We need plumbers and builders with fewer skills, but what we describe as functional literacy – the ability to read simple instructions so as to be able to employ simple but novel techniques.

The products that builders and plumbers come into contact with are manufactured to incorporate more sophisticated technology, and require less and less plumbing and building skills and more and more general reading skills. A plumber's job looks more like a librarian's job than it did a 100 or even 50 years ago. And this is not only the case for plumbers and builders. The mechanic who services my car tells me that he attends night classes in order to keep abreast of the computer-based diagnostic systems that are used in every car repair shop. The mechanic who services my motorcycle tells me that he spends an hour first thing every morning going through his emails to manage the information that is essential for running his business. The mechanic who conducts the government-required test the previously hidden assumptions explicit has been an important process in creating a more open education system. However, we need to understand what the new 'hidden curriculum' is.

The major message that has been put alongside the content of the curriculum is that learning should be easy and entertaining. If pupils and students are not learning, then it must be because the material has not been broken down adequately into its constituent elements, or it has not been properly packaged into the right media for instruction.

Neil Postman (1985) has examined this phenomenon in considerable depth in *Amusing Ourselves to Death*. People have become used to the idea that any information of importance can be passed on in 30 seconds if the presentation is slick enough, as it is in television adverts. Television drama follows the same line, when each hour of viewing has to be self-contained, and does not presume any prior knowledge. 'Series' are designed to present familiar characters, but it must not impair enjoyment if any previous episode has been missed.

This attitude to what it is to be informed has spread progressively from advertisements, to drama, to all kinds of instruction and learning. Literature is short stories. History is made up of one hour documentaries. Biology is an hour of watching entertaining animals, and so on.

Where there is some doubt that the attention of the audience may be wandering, extrinsic motivation will be added in, in the form of a phone-in competition or participative voting scheme. There is no suggestion that learning should be of interest for its own sake.

And while we have been concentrating on the 'delivery' of the curriculum, we have done nothing to change its content, even though its content has been becoming progressively less relevant to the young people in formal education. Perhaps a few examples would make the distinction clearer.

Over the course of studying physics myself, and of training to be an engineer, I developed some quite clear opinions that were based upon what I had learned and the ways of thinking that I had adopted. For example, I had formed a quite clear opinion about which kind of nuclear power stations I felt comfortable to be near. I frequently went sailing at or near the Essex School Sailing Centre at Bradwell on the Blackwater. This necessarily meant spending some days in clear view of the power station at Bradwell. Since this is an old magnox power station I never had any real reason for concern over the reliability of the power station, and I felt quite safe. In contrast with this, I would not have felt happy to be close to a pressurized water reactor, the kind that led to the unfortunate leakage of nuclear material at Three Mile Island.

The judgement is based upon the engineering properties of materials. Magnox power stations use gas to cool the nuclear core of the reactor, while pressurized water reactors use water, as the name implies. In normal working conditions, gas is not very dense, has fairly poor powers of conducting heat and is, as a result, a relatively poor coolant. In contrast with this, water is dense, conducts heat better than a gas, and is a very good coolant, as its use as a coolant in the majority of motor car engines demonstrates. Add to this the fact that a gas-cooled power station has to be a sealed system, as car engines do not, and the clear choice for the coolant of a power station would appear to be water.

However, in assessing engineering systems, one has to take into account likely modes of failure, as well as normal working conditions. For a nuclear power station, an easily imaginable scenario of failure involves an unexpected rise in the temperature of the core of the reactor.

Gas may be a poor coolant, but as the temperature rises its properties as a coolant improve, since its ability to conduct heat depends on the movement of the gas molecules, and this is increased by the higher temperature. The most likely scenario for reactor failure, therefore, includes a self-correcting mechanism, in which the coolant improves to meet the need. In contrast with this, water, when it gets hotter, even pressurized water, is in danger of boiling and turning into steam at higher temperatures, which would bring about a dramatic, not to say catastrophic, deterioration of its properties as a coolant. In such a case, the reactor would not merely be overheated, but the coolant would lose any capacity to reduce the temperature, and the scene would be set for a runaway failure in which increased temperature would lead to a vicious cycle, as it did at Chernobyl.

I therefore form the view that, in spite of the fact that water cooled reactors are cheaper to build and more efficient to run than a gas cooled reactor, because of the way they are likely to behave in an emergency, I am quite happy to live near a gas-cooled reactor but would be uncomfortable living close to a pressurized water reactor. This is not, of course, the view of the matter that is taken by politicians and businessmen who are more concerned about the day-to-day costs of running the plant.

Not that I spent any time at all when I taught physics for a living teaching anything that connected with such political decisions. That would be science that would relate to the life of students as citizens. The curriculum, having been designed for those who might become professional scientists, focused on the properties of materials, but never linked the information to everyday concerns. I never taught about greenhouse gases, global warming, solar energy or any of the other myriad topics that would have interested my pupils. I taught the physics curriculum, and expected my pupils to find their own way of making it relevant, if they could.

However, a second example should also make clear that not all efforts to move the curriculum towards the everyday are successful. Many years ago, as part of the programme of enriching pupils' experience, I took a party of physics students to an open day at the University of Cambridge Faculty of Engineering. The pupils were introduced to the idea that reinforced concrete design could be of interest, by picking the example, from the multitude of possibilities, that they might be involved in designing the containment vessel for a nuclear reactor. Clearly, such three dimensional design would be complex, so the pupils were shown demonstrations on reinforced concrete beams, and invited to make the extension for themselves, by analogy, to the containment vessel.

The demonstrations involved testing reinforced concrete beams to destruction, where the concrete beams were all of the same size (and therefore contained the same amount of concrete), but where the amount of steel reinforcement was increased (and possibly, although I forget the exact details, pre-stressed). The tests showed that, up to the point of first cracking of the beams, the more reinforcement there was in the beams, the stronger they were.

And that was that. The young people were left with the view that the more steel reinforcement was put in concrete, the stronger the concrete was, and that the engineers knew exactly what they were doing when designing containment vessels.

I came away from those demonstrations deeply disturbed. It seemed to me that if the open day was designed to show the real life dilemmas that face engineers, and through them citizens, then an opportunity had been missed. As I indicated in my previous example, an engineer should consider at least two scenarios in designing a structure – everyday use and failure. Since the demonstrations had only considered everyday use they were, at best, partial.

Reinforced concrete can fail in one of two ways; the steel can stretch and fail, or the concrete can be crushed in compression. For obvious reasons, the less reinforcement is in the concrete, the more likely the beam is to fail by the steel stretching, and for the eventual failure to be in the steel. Conversely, the more reinforcement is in the concrete, the more likely it is that the concrete will fail and the steel will remain intact. There would seem to be little difference, except that steel and concrete fail in very different ways. Steel fails relatively slowly in these circumstances, requiring progressively greater loads to produce further distortions. As a result, where the steel fails there are likely to be obvious cracks in the structure, and considerable warning of impending failure. Concrete, on the other hand, tends to fail suddenly; once part of the structure starts to crumble, increased load is placed on the remaining parts, which can then be subject to a runaway failure. Over the past decades a number of reinforced concrete structures have indeed collapsed extremely precipitately, with tragic results.

Overall, the pupils came away from the open day in engineering with the impression that reinforced concrete structures could be made stronger by the inclusion of more reinforcement. In fact, however, I would prefer to live near an under-reinforced containment vessel than an over-reinforced containment vessel, for exactly the same reason as I would prefer to live near a gas-cooled nuclear reactor than a water-cooled nuclear reactor. In both cases the former will be cheaper to build and run, but would give almost no warning of an impending failure. This is actually the decision that needs to be made, and it is a political and economic decision rather than an engineering decision.

I am not normally very keen on the use of the word 'authentic' to describe educational settings, but I think that in this case it is the best word to describe the need. If the curriculum is to be changed in a way that addresses the need of the citizen to understand questions of the day, then it needs to be done in an authentic way. An inauthentic presentation, which essentially removes the critical elements of the discussion, does more harm than good.

This has been a long diversion into the way in which the curriculum, in this case the science curriculum, could be made more relevant to the needs of the average citizen rather than the future specialist in science and engineering. The main purpose of that diversion has been to show how little has actually been done. If anything, teachers have been discouraged from introducing anything that might have overtones of political controversy.

A good example of this has been in sex education. When I was teaching in schools in the 1970s, science teachers were discouraged from teaching anything but the physical arrangements of sex. This knowledge was to be imparted in a 'clinical' way, in the absence of relationship education. By and large, this has now been recognized as a complete failure, and there is a move to teach sex education together with relationship education. However, there are still quite strong social and political pressures about what kind of relationship education can legitimately be included, and in any event, teachers are not always being given the support that is needed to develop approaches that they are comfortable with. The possible outcome, and I am by no means suggesting that it is the necessary outcome in all cases, is an inauthentic education, which cuts out any difficult dilemmas and critical examination. If we wish to give young people an authentic introduction to relationship education, we cannot presume that they will always come to the conclusions that we wish them to.

Teachers (and not only teachers) are rather prone to believe that process and outcome are inextricably linked, and that if we teach young people about the methods that we favour, the learners will come to the same conclusions as we wish them to. Rather similar results are produced when we try to impose democracy, on the assumption that those who have democracy imposed upon them will come to the same conclusions as we would. We have all too many examples of the fact that this rarely works, and it does not work because it is an inauthentic approach. Young people in compulsory education deserve better.

This examination of the question of how the curriculum could be reformed has indicated, I hope, how little has been done to convert the curriculum into a mass curriculum. Fundamentally, the curricula of different subjects are selected and evaluated in terms of the professional needs of specialist groups. If there is any doubt about that, it would quickly be dispelled by looking a the membership of the panels that produced the subject benchmarks for university degree subjects on behalf of the Quality Assurance Agency in Higher Education (QAA). The slow and halting curriculum reforms that have taken place have been introduced by those same specialists as a way to manage the image of their profession in the eyes of young people, and have not been an authentic attempt to address the critical dilemmas that face their profession. We have moved from a selective system of education to a mass system of education, but we have retained a selective curriculum, and not made very much effort to produce a mass curriculum.

This failure to reform the curriculum has been serious enough. It is easy enough to engage young people in the pressing issues of the day outside school; global warming, recycling, world poverty, war, disaster and famine all attract the attention of huge numbers of young people, who are generally agreed to be enthusiastic and idealistic when faced with the problems of the day. Yet in school, subjects which should inform discussion on these pressing questions are taught in a way that fails to engage more than a tiny minority of pupils and students. A few students will study a subject because they are literally inspired by it and wish to know more. A few more will tolerate it because they can see that it is the key to a future profession to which they aspire. A few more will study it because study is not entirely uncongenial, and in any case continuing to study is easier than facing the social stigma of dropping out. But the vast majority of learners will regard study as a tedious necessity that has little or nothing to do with their everyday lives, either now or in the future. And it is difficult to see that they are entirely wrong.

However, the failure to reform the content of the curriculum may not be the greatest shortcoming of the way pupils are taught in our schools and colleges at the moment. Far worse is the idea that the curriculum is fine, and young people would find it interesting if it were only presented in a more dynamic and entertaining way. This is not an attitude that is restricted to education. Which of us has not heard a politician defending a dreadful policy with the words: 'We have the right policy and the public will recognize that if we can only get our message across'. This idea that an unpalatable message can be made palatable by improving the media of communication is the ultimate step towards the inauthentic.

Again, let me stress, I am not opposed to educational technology, or making lessons more interactive, or greater openness in the learning outcomes and the criteria that will be used to assess them. Nor am I opposed to the introduction of interactive whiteboards in schools, or the use of online resources and virtual learning environments. All of these seem to me to be valuable ways of enhancing the student experience. Their presence or absence, however, is not what is wrong with education. What is wrong with education is that we are teaching the wrong things. We are teaching young people for the future that we think that they will have, not for the present that they do have. And they rebel against it.

They rebel against it in increasing numbers. They do not wish to be in classrooms doing the things that we impose upon them. And when they will not sit still for that curriculum, we call them 'hyperactive', and we consider it appropriate to medicate them into submission.

This, of course, brings me back to my main theme, as to whether we should expect to be able to use drugs to improve the extent to which young people can absorb the current curriculum. We need to ask ourselves whether absorption of the current curriculum, whatever that may happen to be at the time, is really the criterion of 'smarter' that we wish to employ. Those whose intellectual life we claim to admire, from Newton to Einstein via Faraday, from Shakespeare to Joyce via Austen, from da Vinci to Bacon via van Gogh, have always been those who have broken the mould, who have rebelled against what they saw before them. As George Bernard Shaw observed, 'All progress depends upon the unreasonable man', and he should doubtless have added, 'and woman'.

'Smarter', therefore, needs to be given more of a social context, and we need to recognize that an ability to succeed in our current curriculum may not be the most effective measure of performance. We have changed our society dramatically. We have pushed individual rights to the fore, and we have increased mechanisms for opening decisions of every kind for examination. We should hardly be surprised that the authority of the teacher has diminished. Indeed, we should hardly be disappointed that the authority of the teacher has diminished. It may be a good thing that children, along with everybody else in society, are less willing to take the authority of people on trust, simply because of the position that they occupy. We cannot expect that we can turn back that trend with increased punishment or with drugs. What we need to be thinking about is how to move forward. What would education look like if we were designing it from scratch today? Focusing on sub-issues, such as the chronic failure of a minority to adapt to what we provide, or the effectiveness of the presentation of archaic material, distracts us from that key question. Treating those who reject our education system as if they were malfunctioning is part of the problem, not part of the solution.

We know that young people can be very idealistic, and show commitment to issues ranging from climate change to animal protection. And we know that a person who has shown commitment, to anything at all from angling to zoology, will go to almost any lengths to satisfy their curiosity about the subject they are interested in. It is, or should be, a source of shame on the part of educationists that they cannot devise curricula in such a way as to take advantage of the natural idealism and inquisitiveness of young people. But part of the problem is that, so long as we think of education in material terms, and as a process of transmitting information from teacher to taught, we will always regard problems as being the result of faulty reception, and not as being rooted in the nature of what we are trying to sell.

Chapter 8

Two Different Approaches to Learning

This chapter will compare and contrast the two approaches to intelligence and learning: the constructivist and the medical. It will identify major differences in ways of thinking about educational settings, but will also highlight differences in the action required in specific circumstances.

Carol Dweck (1999) presents two different approaches to the understanding of intelligence. She divides people into those that she describes as 'entity theorists' and 'incremental theorists'. Entity theorists believe that intelligence is something that a person is born with, and it does not change much through life. Intelligence is a 'thing' that people either have, or do not have. In contrast with this, incremental theorists believe that intelligence is not something that one owns, but is a faculty that one exercises. Moreover, it develops with use, so that one may become more intelligent through hard work and concentrated effort. In this context, however, 'theorist' does not imply some abstract or isolated process conducted in the academy. Each of us has a theory about our own intelligence and how we learn, and it will affect the way that any learner approaches a topic.

Dweck argues that at any specific level of education – say primary or early secondary – there may not be any obvious difference between the performance of entity theorists and incremental theorists. Both may be quite capable of learning and show competence in the areas of study where they are working. The difference only becomes apparent when the learners who hold these different views of their own processes move on to more difficult work. At that point, if the work becomes difficult, the entity theorist is likely to conclude that they are not smart enough for this more difficult work, that they have reached the limit of their potential, that they have developed as far as they can, and that they should probably give up. Incremental theorists are likely to see this as an opportunity for growth, to recognize that the fact that it is getting difficult shows that they are learning something new, and redouble their efforts. Dweck's book recounts many incidents of this division, some of which are really quite touching.

Of course, there is always the possibility that the entity theorist will find the transition easy, and will carry on working alongside incremental theorists effectively, and there will be no real difference between the two, until the next step up in challenge takes place, at which more incremental theorists will put in an increased effort and more entity theorists will give up and drop out. Eventually, the entity theorist will reach a limit when they feel the effort that is needed is too much.

We can understand this quite easily in terms of Vygotsky's notions of how we learn. We start with a higher mental activity, such as memory or focusing attention, and we have some skill in it, which we might regard as due to a natural capacity. We can then learn additional techniques and tools which are driven by, or managed with, cultural signs and symbols that we learn from the culture that we are embedded in and from teachers, playmates and colleagues who surround us. Once we have learned these 'artificial' supplements to our natural abilities, we incorporate them into our everyday practice until they become practically indistinguishable from the 'natural' abilities that we started with. At which point we will be ready to start learning about the new techniques which build upon those we have already acquired. In this way the higher mental functions, although not the basic operation of the brain, can be extended with, Vygotsky believed, no necessary limit.

As will be noted, Vygotsky believed that one was born with something, some basic reflex mechanism, but that that system could be developed and extended by the addition of culturally shaped tools, effectively increasing the intelligence of the individual and the group. In order to be an entity theorist, one has to believe that only the basic functions that one is born with are important, and that the addition of any new ability is peripheral, and does not have any fundamental effect on one's intelligence.

To put this another way, the entity theorist believes that the basic brain function is what is important in intelligence, while the incremental theorist believes that what is important is what is added to the basic brain function through learning.

It should be very clear, even from this brief description, that Vygotsky was an incremental theorist, and was critical of those fellow scientists and contemporaries who were entity theorists. But it should also be clear that incremental theorists and entity theorists will differ greatly in their approach to brain science and what it can tell us that is relevant to the understanding of higher mental functions. Since entity theorists think that intelligence is something that we are born with and cannot do much about, they will think that intelligence is a physical characteristic of the brain, and that brain scans are an opportunity to study that entity. They will think that brain scans that tell us that this or that part of the brain shows increased activity when the subject is thinking about mathematics, or history, or is visualizing a beautiful place, are telling us something important about the mental processes that are going on.

The incremental theorist, on the other hand, thinks that intelligence can change over the period of one's life, and thinks that cultural tools that are acquired over time can help develop mental skills. But the proper place to look for cultural and social signs and symbols is a library, not a brain scan. That is to say, for the incremental theorist, what is being thought, the content of thought, is more important than the mechanism of thought, and that will never show up in a brain scan, no matter how refined brain scans may become.

So, in a curious twist, the entity theorist, who believes that intelligence is fixed, and there is not much that we can do about it, is more likely than the incremental theorist to believe that a drug that operates on the physical performance of the brain will make him or her more intelligent, while the incremental theorist will think that a drug operates at a level which has hardly any bearing on intellect. The entity theorist will point to the effects of alcohol, tiredness and stress and argue that the physical underperformance leads to poor intellectual performance. The incremental theorist will indicate that that the effects of alcohol, tiredness and stress can be overcome by purely mental techniques, at least to some extent, or when it is not possible to overcome the effects, it is at least possible to recognize the effects, and put off any important decisions until one is sober, well-rested and relaxed. The entity theorist, therefore, is more likely to believe in the efficacy of a 'smart drug' which will improve his or her performance.

While Dweck's description of entity theorists and incremental theorists is, superficially, even-handed, there can be little doubt that her intention is to persuade readers that the incremental theorists are right, and the entity theorists have not understood the nature of the activity that they are engaged in. The question remains, therefore, as to why it should be that the entity theory of intelligence is so dominant. It is dominant in the sense that the majority of individuals appear to believe it. But it is also dominant in the sense that major intellectual and professional organizations seem to endorse it, at least implicitly. The idea that the physical results of brain science will provide profound insights into the functioning of the mind and hence have implications for the educational process is so commonplace as to be near universal. The review of smart drugs by the Academy of Medical Sciences (2008) came to a similar conclusion to the review of literature on brain science by the Teaching and Learning Research Programme (TLRP, 2007). In essence this conclusion was that brain science has, to date, provided very little of practical benefit in the way of guidance for educational processes, but it is very likely to in the near future.

This faith that 200 years of the history of science is about to be reversed, and the hope that the precise location and physical nature of a thought is about to be revealed, appears to be absolutely resilient in the face of repeated failure, and the rejection first of phrenology, then of subsequent efforts to localize specific mental activities to particular parts of the brain. Not only do individuals continue to believe it, but the policy positions of professional bodies seem to be in accord with it, and apparently even the structure and organization of our education system depends on it.

The signal that tells an entity theorist that they are getting close to achieving their full potential is that thinking becomes more difficult. Therefore, for the entity theorist to succeed, the most important thing is that they should never face a condition that they think is difficult. Certainly they should never face failure, which is likely to damage their self-confidence and prevent them from advancing. And so we structure our educational system to bolster the self-esteem of every individual. Self-esteem, self-confidence and an unshakeable faith in one's own capabilities are the most important characteristics that we can develop, because anything else spells doom and failure for the entity theorist.

The result is that we have a growing population who are increasingly certain of their own competence in spite of clear evidence to the contrary. We see people who clearly have no understanding of the extent of their own talents, or lack of them, who put themselves forward on the basis of their own self-perception. We see them in talent shows, on quiz shows, in karaoke bars. I am a competent member of a pub quiz team, a reasonable karaoke performer at a family party, can tell an amusing anecdote to friends, but would never imagine putting myself forward to appear on television displaying any of these talents. It just makes it inexplicable to me why there are so many people who do not have a realistic assessment of the fact that they are going to be eliminated from any competition at a very early stage.

One is reminded of Winston Churchill's description of Clement Attlee, the Labour Prime Minister who succeeded him: 'He is a modest man: but then he has so much to be modest about'. When we are faced on all sides by so much to be modest about, it might be refreshing if it were coupled on occasion with a measure of modesty. But our society, and our education system, is built upon the necessity of building up people's self-esteem, of developing their self-confidence. The idea that anything is worth working for has to a very great extent disappeared.

In that sense, the development of smart drugs is on much the same basis as the development of an appetite suppressant, of nicotine patches, of Viagra tablets and of dietary supplements. Anything that we wish to achieve should be achievable without effort, without exercise, without will power and above all without waiting.

In contrast with this, the incremental theorist thinks that effort will improve performance, that learning something does not simply mean the acquisition of something new, but it means changing the person who learns. What the incremental theorist needs is not a boost to his or her self-confidence. They need clear, reasoned evaluations of how they match up against external criteria. In time, through watching how their peers and teachers assess their performances, they will learn how to apply those same criteria to themselves. They will internalize standards of judgement, and criteria for success, and in the process they will gain the tools for managing further self-improvement.

What should be clear is that people should all be incremental theorists, but that being an entity theorist offers a simple let-out, an excuse for not making any effort: 'I am the way that I am, and there is nothing that I can do about it'. The extremes to which this view is taken can perhaps be seen in one of the areas described as suitable for the development of drug treatment, as described in the report of the Academy of Medical Sciences (2008). It may be possible to develop drugs to erase memory selectively, so that, for example, a memory of a serious trauma could be removed. The notion that we might become better people through our experiences, including our traumas, has obviously never occurred to many entity theorists.

Our society is increasingly structured for entity theorists who want achievement to be part of their natural entitlement, without actually having to work for it. Once upon a time we used to eat food. But now we eat fibre and vitamins and fats (though only in the smallest possible quantities) and yoghurts to ease our digestion in the face of the fact that we have stopped eating food. Everything is supposed to have a quick fix, and nothing is supposed to require any effort. And that includes our education system.

There are, of course, major exceptions to this trend, and the most obvious happens when people leave their workplace and embark upon a hobby. And then an extraordinary transformation takes place. A child who will not devote any effort at all to learning arithmetic, will devote endless hours to learning about the history of his or her local football team or favourite pop group. A man who will expend the minimum of mental effort at work will gladly devote hours of time and study to the performance of racehorses, the tying of a trout fly, or the detail of historical army uniforms. If you want to see people functioning in areas where they attach no importance to the expenditure of time, effort or money, then you need to see them when they are playing.

This distinction between working and playing is so sharp in our culture that children recognize the difference at a very early age. The distinction is not about how difficult the thought processes are, or how colourful the educational apparatus is or how the furniture is arranged. The difference is about who decides what the activity is that is to be the focus of attention. If I decide, it is play. If you decide, it is work. Or possibly if you decide, and I agree voluntarily to your choice, we might play together. But if we decide to play together and I am not happy with your choice, believe me that it will not be long before I communicate what hard work it is playing this game.

This should put into perspective the idea that children learn best through play. Children learn best through play because all of us learn best through play. We are playing when we have chosen the activity ourselves, or have voluntarily bought into somebody else's choice, and at that moment all considerations of saving effort or doing things in the easiest way are discarded. At that point self-improvement, not self-esteem, becomes the most important thing to us. We want to be better performers at tiddlywinks or rounders or bridge or whatever it is that we have decided to play at. A few of us are lucky enough to have jobs where we can get along by playing. The rest of us are gardeners who have to earn a living by delivering the mail, or anglers who have to sit in an office all week to earn the right to play at the weekends.

Playing is what we do for its own sake, and we would do anyway, irrespective of incentives, pay, coercion or instruction. Playing is when we can really start to learn. We may acquire some information because we are obliged to do so, but we only really learn in play. That is not, of course, to say that playing requires no effort. Playing may well require more effort of all kinds than anything else that we do, as the examples above make clear. Nor is playing necessarily aimless or undirected. Play can be extremely purposeful. The main criterion for play is that I have chosen to do it myself.

It is perhaps worth noting that this is not a particularly novel perspective on education. In fact, it may even be the majority opinion among educationists. Montessori is today perhaps best remembered for introducing a relatively strict regime of activities for young children. It should, however, be remembered that her method of education did not start out that way. Montessori argued that it was possible to teach a child anything, so long as the teacher did not try to engage the child's reason. To that end her goal was to design, on scientific principles, an environment in which the child could choose their own activities, and in the process the child would educate himself or herself. The success of this approach rested upon the ability to design apparatus in such a way that the child would play with it, and in play be obliged to learn, especially through the self-training of the senses. The most important element of Montessori's scheme, however, was the removal of adults who could direct children as to how they should play. The educational principles should be embodied in the apparatus, not in any supplementary instructions.

Whether Montessori was right about not trying to engage the reason of the young child or not, I am sure that this cannot be a principle for higher levels of education. In higher education particularly, what we are trying to develop is a critical self-awareness, an ability to manage one's own memory and attention and apply reference criteria. And this may also be the case in secondary education. However, what is clear is that we should make every effort to ensure that the learner, of whatever age, disengages that part of their reason that counts the cost, in time or effort, of the activity in which they are engaged. And that is done by linking learning with play.

As I have noted elsewhere, we have moved away from a society where people of whatever age are prepared to take somebody else's word for it, whatever 'it' may be. We question authority in all its forms. And this is seen to lead to a deterioration of discipline, in our schools and elsewhere in our society. But we need to be clear about what it is that has been lost. We have lost the sense that one person ought to be able to impose an activity on another. That is true in schools as it is in other institutions and outside. In schools, this makes life more difficult for teachers. It is no longer possible to give young people work in the expectation that they will do it for no other reason than that it has been given. And that sense of discipline is never likely to be regained. It should, however, be noted that what has been lost is not the part of school life that was devoted to learning. The opposite is true. What has been lost is the part of school life that is antagonistic to learning.

What we now need to seek are new ways of organizing learning so that it is tolerable for both learners and teachers, and so that it is enjoyable and fruitful for those who wish to play. Over the past 50 years, while most of society has been changing in a direction that undermines imposed, external discipline, successive governments have been making concerted efforts to reinforce discipline and control in educational institutions. From imposed external criteria to specification of curriculum content, from preferred methods for teaching reading, writing and arithmetic to published measures of success, governments have been making every effort to ensure that schools are places of work, not places of play.

Talking about 'time on task' or 'efficiency' is a discourse about work. As soon as one accepts such language as appropriate to the school, then one has stopped talking about school as an educational institution and started talking about it as an instrument of something else, quite possibly coercion and social control, but definitely not education. What we need is much less efficiency and more time 'wasted'. The likelihood is that more learning would take place in such an atmosphere.

Education is being driven in the wrong direction. Traditional models of managing people are ceasing to work, and for reasons that most of us would approve. People are more aware of their rights, more willing to stand up for themselves, less willing to take things on trust, and so on. Schools are being asked, not only to move in the opposite direction, but to move so far in the opposite direction that they can compensate for all the changes that have happened in society outside schools. This cannot be done. Schools need to find a new direction.

I am not exactly sure what such a direction would be like. But what is clear is that everybody needs to become an incremental theorist. Everybody needs to understand that they can develop and grow throughout life, through the much vaunted lifelong learning process, and in doing so each person can create the major work of their life – him- or herself. And then each person should be encouraged to play at that project.

There is nothing quite so corrosive to that idea as the notion that a smart drug might produce some valuable effects. What is important in higher mental functions is that which is furthest from the purely physical connections of neurons. If smart drugs can have an effect, they can only affect the least important aspects of our thought. To believe otherwise is to undermine the notion that people can improve themselves through effort and through adopting mental frameworks and schema that change the way they see the world and themselves.

The problem that we face is that smart drugs may have a huge effect on education, not by any physical effect that they may have on people who take them. The real problem with smart drugs is that the idea of them may shape the way that we think about what education is. Smart drugs alone cannot have this effect. But the fact that we think it likely that smart drugs might work underlines the fact that we are thinking about education in a completely unhelpful way.

Chapter 9

Discipline and Respect

We have heard a lot about the 'respect agenda' and when problems with young people are discussed, especially in the popular media, the solution is often linked with a lack of discipline, or a need to reintroduce a notion of discipline. It therefore seems appropriate to examine the words 'respect' and 'discipline' in some detail.

One of the most obvious problems with the two words is that they come in at least two major forms – directed towards oneself and directed towards others. For example, respect can mean either self-respect or, more commonly in the context of the 'respect agenda', be linked to a call for increasing the respect that young people show to others, and most particularly to a return to a traditional value of respect for one's elders. The fact that the word has those two meanings often, also, leads to an elision whereby it is supposed that if only we could impose a regime where children were forced to show respect for their elders or for those in authority, then they would, in some miraculous way, learn self-respect, or conversely, if we could in some way boost their self-respect, they would learn respect for others.

In a similar way, 'discipline' covers both self-discipline and an externally imposed regime of punishments and rewards, and apart from the fact that the same word covers both, there is very little to connect the two concepts. The idea that military discipline, either in the form of national service or a boot camp, might in some way develop self-discipline in those who have never known it before, seems to be the result of this cruel pun.

In addition, 'discipline' describes a structure of knowledge divided into strands that suit the professional academic very well, but which are of limited relevance to those of us who have to use knowledge however we can to solve everyday problems. In the latter case, whether a specific piece of knowledge is history, geography or mathematics is of less importance to us than whether it can be used to produce a desirable result. But the idea that knowledge comes naturally formed into disciplines is extremely deep-rooted, and leads to a subsidiary pun which cuts short much of our discussions of curriculum reform; what young people need is discipline, or an introduction to the disciplines, and therefore they need to be introduced to the core subjects, or disciplines, in schools. Again, by a process of elision, it is relatively easy to assume that children need certain basic disciplines, such as literacy and numeracy, without actually thinking about why they need either. The idea of a discipline also puts the content of a subject area out of dispute, and wraps it up in a bundle, decided by experts, which is very difficult to reconsider. 'Numeracy' becomes one of those motherhood and apple pie concepts, which it is very difficult to argue against. Obviously, children need to be numerate, but it is not at all clear that they need to know the proof of Pythagoras' Theorem or be able to solve simultaneous equations. Or, at least, it is not at all obvious that all children need to know these things. But the idea of a discipline in this sense allows us to wrap up all mathematics in one package, and assume that everybody needs it all.

On the other hand, it would be foolish to suggest that there is no connection between respect which we show to others and the self-respect which we develop in the process of education. But there is not an automatic or necessary connection, and the relationship needs to be teased out in more detail. In particular, what is needed to link the two is a theory of learning. Vygotsky has offered such a theory.

Vygotsky argued that from our earliest experience we discover that other people try to manage our behaviour using language. The word, 'No' is one of the first expressions that we may hear, and it is a clear indication that others expect to be able to intervene in the gap between our desires and our actions by using language. Similarly, we learn at a very early age that we can have an effect on the behaviour of others through the use of language, or perhaps even before language through screams and/or smiles. Screaming gets us fed, or picked up, or changed, depending upon the circumstances.

However, the greatest discovery that we make is that we can come to control our own behaviour through the use of language. We were born with certain reflexes, such as the response to turn towards a loud noise. With time we come to replace a loud noise with paying attention to a particular person's voice, and then to the sound of our own name. The external stimulus which attracts our attention can be made subtler and subtler, and eventually we can use the thought of our own name as a way of managing our attention. Thus, what started out as an external process, where my mother showed me how she could control what I did, came to be an internal mechanism by which I could self-manage.

Vygotsky argued that this process is typical of learning. Our higher mental functions, by which Vygotsky means those which make us specifically human as opposed to animal, and which include focusing attention, managing memory, planning and critical evaluation, start out as relationships between people. However, learning involves two cycles, an interpersonal cycle, in which we come to understand about the possibility of some new learning in a social setting, and an intrapersonal cycle in which that new possibility is internalized.

When I was a child we used to solve crossword puzzles as a family. My father would read out clues from the newspaper, and my mother, and I suppose initially only my mother, used to offer suggestions as to possible answers. Eventually, by listening to this conversation over a very long period of time, one came to understand how a cryptic clue was constructed, and why the answers that my parents thought were correct were correct. Those standards, which started out as observations about a public conversation, came to be internalized, so that I would know whether an answer that was suggested was correct or not. Eventually, I would have suggestions of my own, and I would be able to evaluate whether those suggestions were good suggestions or wild guesses, because I had internalized the standards of judgement. But I also knew, as the youngest person involved in the exercise, that I was unlikely to be the fastest person producing a response to any clue. So what started as a social exercise, quite explicitly worked through in public, where somebody who suggested an answer was expected to be able to justify it in a rational way, came to be internalized as a way of thinking about and playing with words. And from time to time I still solve crosswords on my own.

But, perhaps more importantly, among those values that were put on public offer in that family setting, I did not choose only to internalize a tendency to solve crosswords. There were other values which I chose to internalize along with that. A love of words was one, and a playfulness over how words were constructed, together with a close attention to the meaning of strange words and a concern over accuracy in spelling would have been those that were most closely associated with the process of solving crosswords.

But there were other, still more general, or transferable, skills or values which went along with the strictly verbal skills. As the youngest member of the family I learned that I could not compete, or was not competing, on a level playing field. If I was the first to solve one clue in a whole crossword, then I was doing very well. My father would solve 70 per cent of the clues, my mother another 20 per cent, my brothers a small and growing number of clues, and not much was left for me. And with time, I came to understand that my father was not simply better at crosswords than the rest of us, but that it gave him a distinct advantage that he was reading out the clues for the rest of us. In the first place, he had 'advanced notice' of the clue, and therefore more time to solve it, since he read it before we heard it. In addition, he could see the frame where the words had to fit, and being able to visualize the words also helps. But in addition, I was solving crosswords with people who were older and more knowledgeable than I was. So I learned to develop my own standards – if my brother solved five clues, that was good for him, but if I solved only one, that was good for me. I do not know whether that was a good thing or a bad thing, but it lives with me still in a reduced urge to be directly competitive, or at least competitive for the sake of being competitive.

I have chosen to review this example at some length because it seems to me to illustrate some of the features of Vygotsky's theory that are crucial to understanding how we learn. This learning was not a process of developing habits. Only on very rare occasions would one meet the same clue twice, in which case memory would serve to produce a solution. What one was learning were the rules for solving crosswords, how the clue has to relate to the solution, giving, in part, a clue to the meaning of the whole word, and in other parts perhaps enable the solver to construct the word from parts. In the end, there had to be a solution that was publicly explicable and intelligible. Those public standards were eventually internalized by each of us, so that we knew when we were on the right track.

But this also relates to the issues of discipline and respect, and the connections between the social and personal meanings of those words. There is a discipline in solving crossword puzzles – one cannot simply dream up solutions that fit in the crossword grid. But that discipline was and is an integral part of the activity. If you do not like the rules, you do not solve crossword puzzles, and no moral value attaches to those who choose to waste their time on crossword puzzles and those who choose to waste their time in other ways. But once a person has chosen the activity, certain disciplines follow as part of that process. My parents did not set out to impose discipline upon us. I suppose that they might have told us to go and play elsewhere if we were too noisy and were distracting them from concentrating on the puzzle, but I do not remember that. The discipline and the concentration arose directly from the activity.

I suppose that my father did enforce the discipline of the crossword in one sense. He had to write the solutions in the grid, and therefore it was he who had to be convinced that an answer was correct. If he was so convinced, he accepted the solution and wrote it down. If he was not so convinced, he suspended judgement (normally until we had some more letters in the grid) and did not write it down. But in a sense that was not arbitrary; it was discipline within the structure of a crossword. It was a discipline that was integral to the achievement of the chosen goals which we all understood. We also understood that in the case of disputes, there would be an unambiguous way of resolving those disputes when the following day the newspaper published the completed crossword. And then we could enter into yet another round of discussion, about which clues were good, and which were poor.

Similarly, respect was signalled socially in the first instance. Anybody could make a suggestion as to what the solution to a clue was. If the connection between the clue and the proposed solution was not immediately obvious to everybody present, it was legitimate to ask for an explanation. Anybody could ask for an explanation, and anybody could be asked to give an explanation. No solution was ever accepted or rejected simply on the grounds of who had suggested it. There was an exception to this, when my father solved a clue before he had a chance to read it out, in which case he might simply write it down without making it available for public scrutiny. But there were enough occasions where subsequent answers created difficulties in the grid and such a solution had to be reconsidered to make it clear that no solution was beyond questioning. I will not say that happened often, but it happened enough to make the principle clear.

Thus respect was shown socially by making it clear that everybody's contributions were valued and carefully considered. And this in turn led us to develop our own take on self-respect. I have no idea what the other people present did with the notion of self-respect, but I came to develop a pride in my own thought processes, to give myself credit when I solved a clue but was not quick enough to be the first to suggest the solution, and to be a severe critic of my own suggestions before I put them forward publicly. These values became part of the way that I think about myself, part of the person that I became.

The central point here is that discipline and respect, as they occur within Vygotsky's theory, are related to the exercise of judgement in relation to standards. Those standards start out as public schema, which is how they relate to external discipline and respect. However, each of us who experiences them in a social setting has an opportunity to internalize them and make them part of our own reasoning, which is how they relate to self-respect and self-discipline.

An important contrast needs to be drawn here with the notion of self-esteem, as it is widely used in education. Self-esteem is used to describe that sense of self-value which arises from affirmation. It is unconditional, in the sense that it is not supposed to be related to specific standards, but is supposed to arise from the fact that we are praised, or encouraged, or valued, whatever we do. It leads to the idea that teachers should first and foremost praise any work which is presented to them, and only then suggest one or two possibilities for improvement. And the balance should be very definitely in favour of the praise; I have heard the suggestion that a teacher's marking should consist of 'three stars and a wish' – three points that are picked out for praise and one point where improvement might be sought. This seems to me to be a highly problematic approach to teaching.

Some years ago I was working on a programme where students were invited to assess their own performance. They were developing skills as entrepreneurs, and therefore were also developing skills which normally fall within the remit of other disciplinary areas, such as marketing, web design or consultancy skills. However, they made that self-assessment without being exposed to the standards that other professionals might have exercised, for example in marketing or web design. The result was that their evaluations were generally positive, even when their work fell well below the standard of work that was routinely done by first year undergraduate students who specialized in those areas.

The problem with self-esteem is that it may not be based on any solid foundations. It is better for a person to have an accurate judgement of how they perform than to be confident that their performance is excellent. We see plenty of examples of people who have very high self-esteem, but who are frankly incompetent. And not all of them are politicians.

This led me on to wonder what is involved in applying standards to the evaluation of students' work. And I found the answer in Vygotsky; when I mark work, what I am doing is making my standards of judgement publicly available to my students. Obviously, I make those standards more accessible if I do not simply put a mark on the bottom of their piece of paper, but also provide an explanation of why that mark is appropriate and how their work measures up to those standards.

It is my hope that the students concerned will internalize those standards, and apply them to their subsequent work, so that they can improve and achieve better marks in the future. It is commonly lamented that students will only complete work for which there is a mark, and that all that concerns them is the mark. But this should not be viewed, as it commonly is, that students have turned off onto some wrong path. It is evidence that they have gone half way along the path that we wished them to follow. They have come to the point where they recognize the socially determined nature of the standards that have been applied. However, we need to keep in mind the fact that the true purpose of education is the personal internalization of those standards, so that everybody who works in a field has become self-regulating, and knows when they are doing a good job.

Students, and everybody else, deserve the respect which is shown in an honest and principled evaluation of their work. Nobody can develop an understanding of those standards if they know that any response is going to be made up of three stars and a wish, whatever the quality of the work they produce. The inevitable outcome of such an approach is that they will dismiss the standards as pointless, or will adopt standards that are low and of little value.

In terms of this framework of what marking is for and how standards fit into the process of learning, it is important to recognize how far the commonsense interpretation of values has strayed from a truly educational approach. In public debate, all the emphasis is placed on the standards applied by external assessors – whether that is on SAT scores for schools, GCSE and A-level results, or final degree classifications, as though they represented in some way the final outcome and purpose of education. In fact, they represent only the end of the first, interpersonal cycle of education, whereas the ultimate goal and purpose of education is the internalization of those values which help people become self-managing, self-improving and reflective professionals.

Of course, there may be reasons other than educational reasons for making sure that we accentuate the positive when giving feedback. Some people may be fragile, and if the first sentence of feedback is negative, they may not be able to get past that to hear anything else. Some people may need reassurance that they are likely to succeed in the end, or they may not consider the effort worthwhile. And we may not wish to cause gratuitous offence in the way that we present feedback on performance. But it should be borne in mind that any such considerations are not educational, though they may be good social or therapeutic reasons for tempering the way in which we express ourselves. 'Three stars and a wish' may be a good rule of thumb for making feedback palatable, but it should never be allowed to dominate the more important, educational purpose of making standards clear. By and large, people find it easier to perform well when they know what the criteria for good performance are, and we will not communicate those criteria effectively if we are too concerned to sugar coat any evaluation.

It is worth, at this point, revisiting the question of discipline and respect as normally described. In a widely held view of the issues involved, young people need to learn that actions have consequences, and to this end we need to impose discipline and clear penalties for breaking the rules. To take an example that is current, young people need to understand that carrying a knife can have serious consequences and that, therefore, all cases of knife carrying should be punished by a term in jail. The fact of the matter is that arming oneself with a knife has serious consequences, not the least of which is that the person carrying the knife is more likely to be injured or to injure somebody else, with severe repercussions for all involved.

If we add to that the idea that knife carrying must be punished by jail, we weaken, rather than strengthen, our argument. We add a further, extrinsic consequence of the action, namely jail, a clear indication that we do not think that the intrinsic consequence, of physical harm, is sufficient disincentive. People should not carry knives because knives are dangerous. People should not steal because theft leads to a breakdown of moral values which support society. People should not copy in exams because this removes the effectiveness of the process, which is to help those who are being examined to form a view of their own competence. When we add additional penalties, all we are doing is acknowledging that the consequences are not as dire as we would wish people to believe. We are helping to promote the view that the only crime worth worrying about is being caught.

Of course, we do need to have penalties for breaches of the rules where people are prepared to transgress for personal benefit in spite of the damage this does to other people. However, we should not confuse this with the need, in general and for the broad mass of people, to explain that actions have intrinsic consequences which make them desirable or undesirable. When we hear claims that what young people need is more imposed discipline so that they can learn that their actions have consequences, we need to think very carefully about what the purpose of our actions is.

Discipline which is imposed can only achieve the first part of the learning process; it can make standards available that the learner can, subsequently, if he or she chooses, internalize to regulate their own behaviour. However, if this is done in such a way, and with such emotional overtones, as to make it unlikely that they will choose to internalize those values, this defeats the whole purpose of the process.

To summarize, Vygotsky has argued that we learn through a process which is first social and interpersonal, and secondly internal and intrapersonal. The first can be controlled and managed by peers and teachers, but the latter is entirely within the control of the learner. We can structure a team-building event, provide frameworks for thinking about teamwork, manage experiences, measure outcomes, but the only people who can decide whether or not they should adopt those values for themselves are the people involved, each one for him- or herself.

People are quite extraordinary in being subject at all times to processes of continual feedback. I am not absolutely sure what I will say before I say it, but as I say it I am reflecting on my own reaction to what I have said (How did that sound? Have I overstated my case? Have I made my point forcefully enough?) at the same time as I am getting feedback from other people (Have I lost their attention? Did I notice a slight nod at that point?). And those feedback loops are filtered through a variety of perceptions and remembered experiences, internalized values and ideas of others (What would my teacher have said about this performance? Was that an ethical thing to say?).

Since Vygotsky died, scientists have made huge advances in understanding systems that are non-linear and have multiple feedback loops. They have developed chaos theory, sometimes called complexity theory, to describe the behaviour of such systems. The development of chaos theory arose from the observation, in various spheres of scientific understanding, that some systems did not behave in the way described by Newton; not all systems are as regular as clockwork, nor do they follow a simple path from their starting position. Chaotic systems, such as weather systems, may be dramatically disturbed by slight shifts in their initial conditions. Ironically, it came to be understood that those systems that Newton was supremely successful in describing, planetary systems, may also be chaotic.

Because the development of chaos theory is relatively recent, there is no way of knowing how Vygotsky would have reacted to it. I like to think, however, that he was struggling towards an understanding of people as chaotic systems, and that he would have embraced chaos theory had it been available to him. Chaos theory describes the behaviour of systems that are self-regulating, and use multiple and complex patterns of feedback in that process of self-regulation. This gives rise to patterns of behaviour that follow quasi-regular cycles, or patterns, but which never precisely repeat, and where very small inputs can produce dramatic changes in outcomes. That seems to me to be not a bad account of people, especially people as Vygotsky described them, who make conscious efforts to self-manage by using language and other external cultural symbols to modify their responses to external events. Although, as Vygotsky emphasized, higher mental functions start out as relationships between people, when we internalize them they become our own, and we modify and develop them in unpredictable and unique ways. That which makes us most human is the intentional process of self-management.

I have no idea whether or not we are born with a desire to make sense out of things. What is clear is that making sense of ourselves and our environments very soon becomes a major driving force in everything that we do. And making sense out of things is not at all the same as seeking a causal chain of events. There is no causal chain of events that will make it possible to calculate what I will be doing next Thursday week from where I am today, or my present mood, or my physical condition. It is not possible to work from my attitudes and dispositions today, to work out what my attitudes and dispositions will be tomorrow, and so on through the days until we arrive at next Thursday week. What I will do then will be made sense of, not causally, but in the light of commitments and agreements that I have made, and which, apart from the peculiar circumstance that I have remembered them in order to write about them now, are for the most part put on one side and forgotten.

That process of making sense plays a crucial part in deciding what we will do. It governs our behaviour as human beings.

There are many ways of failing to show respect for other human beings, but one of the most egregious is to ignore the fact that their sense-making is an important part of their motivation and their activity. We show a lack of respect for people when we try to understand them as pieces of machinery, or as animals. When we think that their performance can be effectively managed by giving them incentives, but without giving the credit for reasoning, we show a basic lack of respect. When we act as though people were driven by basic instincts, such as hunger or sex, we treat them as no better than rats. And if we structure our society, our marketing, or modes of exchange and our assumptions on the basis that hunger and sex are the most important things in life, we treat ourselves with a complete lack of respect.

Respect and discipline are important in all aspects of learning. But in a curious Orwellian turn of phrase, respect and discipline come to be counter-educational in many ways. What we often mean by respect and discipline is an unthinking deference to arbitrary authority. We dislike and reject arbitrary authority in many areas of our lives. We do not expect to accept the ruling of a petty bureaucrat or a hereditary ruler. We do not expect to sit still and be lectured by our politicians or our priests. And yet those freedoms which we happily embrace for ourselves we would deny to young people in education. And we are surprised when they will not sit still for the lectures either.

There is a major opportunity here for education to recast itself in a new mould for present-day society. We could recast an education which started from the intrinsic values and benefits of learning, and not from externally imposed notions of discipline and respect. I am not sure exactly what that would look like, but there are some indications in what we have seen so far, and I shall develop them more fully in the next chapter. What is certain is that attempts to impose either respect or discipline externally on young people, without modelling respect and discipline in our own approach to them, is likely to be counter-productive.

There is a connection here between the insistence upon order, and the tendency to think of education in terms of medical models. Medical models imply a range of mental tools that presuppose causation, that test for causation through a series of double-blind experimental methods, and similar 'scientific' approaches, and these in turn are applied to testing the effectiveness of the curriculum. Perhaps we should even stop thinking about curriculum measures, and talk instead of 'educational treatments'. That is to say that medical models are a shorthand for a specific type of supposedly scientific approach which is very difficult to combine with a need to recognize the individuality of learners. I have written elsewhere about the limits of educational theory, and the fact that the models that we choose should leave space for individual difference and free will (Turner, 2004). It should be clear that medical models do not match up to such standards. And it may be worth noting in this context that Vygotsky spoke of the *history* of the development of higher mental functions and not the *science* of that development (Rieber, 1997). We each have unique personal histories, and education should be designed to help that individuality flourish, not constrain it into a scientific mould.

Chapter 10

Whither Education?

Now if we come to look at how education should be shaped, there are a number of messages that need to be taken away. In the first place, we need to note that social and labour market changes have occurred, so that education is seen as important for people who would, in the past, have been excluded from education, or would have excluded themselves.

Economists speak of an S-curve to describe the take-up of innovations; there is a slow take up in the early stages as the more adventurous take it up, followed by a rapid take-up in the middle phase when the innovation has become mainstream, ending in a slow creep towards universality as those least convinced of the benefits of the innovation come on board. This has certainly been the case in education, at least as far as the first two stages of the process were concerned.

Up until the 1950s, the expansion of higher education had been slow, with only a minority of the population being engaged. In the middle of the nineteenth century only lawyers, doctors and priests had needed university education. But in a process that began in the mid to late nineteenth century, and continues today, successive professions and para-professions have placed increasing demands on new entrants to have post-compulsory education as part of their essential preparation. In the USA first and then later in Europe, accountants, engineers, nurses, teachers, psychologists and many associated professions took their place as professions with corresponding programmes of preparation in universities. Even so, the growth in the number of occupations that needed university education was modest compared with the late twentieth century, when a growing proportion of jobs required education at an advanced level, especially with the establishment of the welfare state after 1945.

The result was that in the 1950s the vast majority of those in higher education came from families where at least one parent had experience of higher education, and a commitment to education for social advancement was part of the family tradition.

In contrast with this, by the end of the twentieth century, growing numbers of students in higher education came from families where nobody had previously progressed beyond secondary education. Indeed, this became something of a political slogan. At the same time, primary and secondary education became near universal.

The consequences of this change are clear. In the 1950s through the 1970s, most of those who were in higher education understood what the process was about. They had resources that they had drawn from their families, in terms of attitudes to study and background knowledge. Although nobody had necessarily gone out of their way to teach students how to manage their concentration, how to read critically, or how to structure an argument, those skills had been picked up along the way, almost unconsciously, possibly while solving crossword puzzles on family holidays.

As teachers, therefore, we need to be thinking about how to make explicit those elements that were previously implicit. We need to be teaching how to read critically, and how to structure arguments, but perhaps most importantly, we need to be teaching what education is about altogether. Above all, the purpose of education is to change the person who undertakes it. The conception of education as something that a person receives, or collects, without being substantially changed, is widespread and more or less has the currency of commonsense. However, it is also probably the biggest obstacle to achieving the goals of education, as it minimizes what a person thinks that they have to do to be successful in education.

We have gone some way towards recognizing this change in education, and to make explicit the demands and expectations that a successful education implies. We can see this in attempts to make learning outcomes explicit. For example, in higher education in the UK, under pressure from the QAA, all courses now have explicit learning outcomes. This was a quite deliberate attempt to make information about programmes available for those who do not have an intimate understanding of higher education. There is a limit to how effective this can be in practice. The QAA started from the expressed intention of producing module and programme descriptors that would make that information accessible to students, parents and employers in simple terms, so that a full understanding of what was involved in any specific programme could be grasped. In practice, this has never really worked, because what information people need, and indeed what specific information means to them, depends very much on their prior experience and interests. Consequently, a single document that provides satisfactorily for the information needs of prospective students, parents and employers has proved elusive.

That project of designing a source of information that would make the purpose of education perfectly transparent to 'outsiders' was not a complete success, and the QAA has had to backtrack on it somewhat. However, in principle, the idea that success in higher education should not be based on hidden criteria and on preparation that was more readily available to the middle classes was an extremely positive move.

What has been rather stranger has been the very negative response that this move has had from professional educators and teachers. In general terms, the move to democratize education, to make access more widely distributed, has been depicted in very negative terms by educationists. It has been argued that the efforts to make outcomes explicit have been a two pronged attack to deskill professional teachers and dumb down academic standards.

The negative underpinnings can perhaps be understood in terms of a parallel with Foucault's vision of control in modern society, and his study of prisons. The argument goes that early or medieval societies were maintained by coercion, which at base, or when all else failed, would rely on physical violence, in the form of an armed police or army, to maintain the interests of those who governed.

In contrast with this, in a modern society people are persuaded to self-police, to internalize the values of those they think are watching them, so that explicit violence is unnecessary. Coercion by force is replaced by internalized coercion, which, of course, from the point of view of those who govern society is cheaper and more effective.

And here we come to the irony of the modern, or perhaps post-modern, interpretation of social control; self-management is given a negative meaning. Self-control is part of the hegemonic process whereby the oppression of the working classes is maintained. And within that framework self-regulation, self-restraint and self-management are all negatively construed. Something of the tone of this argument, as it relates to education, can be seen in the work of Baker and Brown (2007). Those authors cite Rose (1999: 149):

> Contemporary individuals are incited to live as if making a *project* of themselves: they are to *work* on their emotional world, their domestic and conjugal arrangements, their relations with employment and their techniques of sexual pleasure, to develop a 'style' of living that will maximise the worth of their existence to themselves. (Stress in the original)

One can gather, from the contemptuous tone, as much as from the words themselves, that Rose regards any sense of self-management as an intrusion into the personal realm by external influences, particularly commercial interests. Separated from that imputation of commercialism, I would say that it was highly commendable that young people in education were encouraged to work on their emotional world, and to think of themselves as their own creation, that they could make themselves into the person that they wish to be. The idea that we do not need to work at our domestic and employment relations, and that whatever is important in life should be instantly available, seems to me to be one of the main shortcomings of modern society and the commercialism that Rose highlights.

Baker and Brown (2007: 146) follow this quote by emphasizing how strong is the link between commercialism and free choice: 'The notion of the self as a free autonomous chooser is closely allied to the sense that post-compulsory education's students are "customers". This has, as we have seen, been embedded in scholarship and policy on the issue.' While there may be a contingent link between some aspects of these two ideas, it seems very far from clear that there is a necessary link, or that any suggestion that students need to exercise choices is a call for rampant commercialism.

However, the fact that self-management and shallow commercialism have been so strongly linked in much of the mainstream literature on education makes it difficult to describe education in Vygotsky's terms, where self-control and self-management are the highest goals to be achieved.

In looking, therefore, for the way forward in education, the first step is to reclaim the idea that the point and purpose of education is to change the self through the addition of mechanisms which increase one's ability to control and manage oneself, and increasing amounts of information and knowledge.

We should perhaps consider two contrasting approaches to education, one in which self-control is seen as the highest aim and end of education, and one in which self-control is considered to be negative, or so hard to achieve as to be irrelevant. In the former, people are changed and empowered by the knowledge and skills that they acquire. A skilled cabinet maker, printer or footballer is a person who has changed him- or herself by devoting him- or herself to the development of a skill, and made the possession of that skill into a way of life. In the latter, more traditional way of thinking about education, a person is pretty much unchanged by his/her encounters with education. People acquire skills and knowledge, and as a result they are more skilful or more knowledgeable, but not much altered otherwise. Since education is about acquiring rather than becoming, external discipline is necessary to manage the learners, who are presumed not to be capable of managing their own development (since not much development is presumed to take place).

In terms of the distinctions that I have been describing throughout this book, the idea that knowledge and skills are things that can be attached to a pre-existing person is rooted in a materialistic view of learning. The person is an entity that new things are added to. In the alternative view, the person approaches education, in Dweck's term, incrementally. They use learning to become different, and hopefully better people. The important aspects of learning are not the things learned, but the processes of self-control that are developed.

Education suffers from a double blow when it comes to seeking a way forward. In the first place it appears that, although people have been thinking about, and studying, education for centuries, there seems to be very little agreement about what is currently known about education. One expert says one thing, another expert says another. We should introduce our children to discipline; we should develop their creativity. They need to develop habits of good spelling early; spelling does not matter so long as they can communicate. And so on.

In the face of this apparent disarray among specialists, everybody has at least some experience of education through their own encounters with it, either positive or negative. In consequence, everybody thinks of themselves as an expert, however naïve or misguided their notions of education are. So it is perhaps surprising that there seems to be something of a consensus on at least one aspect of the mind–body problem among philosophers and psychologists of very different persuasions. As I have indicated, most great thinkers on questions related to education have rejected the notion of materialism and a materialistic understanding of the mind and its operations.

As I mentioned previously, Popper takes a very strong stance against materialism. The essence of his argument is that there is something about our thoughts which is social or external. The critical, scientific community has developed, and can further develop knowledge which he describes as having some kind of external reality.

While I do not particularly care for the word 'reality', that need not be an obstacle to acknowledging that our thoughts are constrained by what we know. We cannot, at will, decide that six is a prime number, or that the Earth is flat.

We set up integrated ways of looking at the world, which certainly may be somewhat arbitrary. But once we have established them, there appear to be non-trivial consequences that we cannot avoid. We set up the rules that tell us how to draw a map of different countries, and how to colour them in, and it appears to us that it ought to be possible to prove that five, and only five, colours are necessary to colour in any map. But the development of that proof takes decades and the dedication of large numbers of mathematicians.

The important point about this is, from my perspective, not whether the proof is 'real', but the fact that it is, in some important way, beyond our control. Certainty that a proof has been produced does not come from any internal conviction, but from a social activity of demonstrating. The proof is valid or not valid, not on the grounds of how strongly it is believed, but on how it is developed logically.

This partial autonomy of the products of our thoughts from the brain processes – or even the mind processes – that produce them, has important consequences for the mind–body problem. Most obviously it means that the content of our thoughts has to be judged by standards which are external, communal and, according to Popper, in some way objective. Even if I follow him only as far as 'external' and 'communal', it means that there is something more to the validity of a thought than just feeling it. It means that the neurons which fire when I think that 6 times 8 is 42 represent a thought which is corrigible by those external standards. There is more to the thought than the firing of a neuron, or even millions of neurons. While drugs and other physical influences may be able to have an influence on whether I think that 6 times 8 is either 42 or 48, nothing can influence which is the right answer, because its rightness lies somewhere beyond my own brain. Standards of judgement, rules of procedure and similar frameworks of judgement are beyond the scope of a materialist interpretation of the mind–body problem.

So it may be surprising to find that this position is not very far from the stance taken by Wittgenstein and Malcolm from a perspective of linguistic philosophy, given that Popper was extremely hostile to linguistic philosophy in all its manifestations.

Wittgenstein argued that a private language, a language used, applied, and importantly verified by only one person, is impossible. We cannot, like Humpty Dumpty in *Alice Through the Looking Glass*, make words mean whatever we choose when we use them. Applying a word in a particular way carries public consequences and implications which cannot be denied. I cannot say that I am in pain, and give a broad, beaming smile. Or, at least, I can lie on one or two occasions, and say that I am in pain, and give a broad beaming smile, but if that is the only way that I ever use the expression you would be entitled to conclude that I did not understand what I was saying. Words have some public existence which has consequences that we cannot fully control.

It may be relevant to ponder one modern area where it is nearly possible to escape from the consequences of our language, in cyberspace. I can 'be' a 15-year-old boy, or even a 15-year-old girl, in an alternative reality. I can learn the slang, follow the interests, create a false persona. But nevertheless, when people who have created false personas in cyberspace meet, they are faced with the consequences of being real bodies, sometimes with tragic consequences.

Interestingly, recent research (Belkin et al., 2008) has indicated that people are more willing to lie in emails than they are when using other media of communication. Modern electronic means of communication introduce new concerns about the authenticity of the person communicating. A similar question arises when using computer simulations in teaching; since a computer can simulate anything, the question of truthfulness arises with particular force. Importantly, emoticons* are not a substitute for body language; they are a deliberate attempt to project an idea of what body language would be, encoded into a different form of language. This truthfulness gap in electronic communication may be very important and may ultimately indicate some kind of limit to electronic communication, a barrier to using only distance education mediated by modern technology.

In contrast with the consensus to be found among philosophers, however, we find an entirely different consensus when we turn our attention to politicians, policy makers, parents and many self-styled experts on education. The idea of promissory materialism, or even current materialism, seems to have achieved something like the status of commonsense. We speak of skills and capabilities as though they could be broken down into their constituent elements and passed on to people. The curriculum should be 'transmitted'. To practise a particular profession, a person must demonstrate that they have this list of competences, as though being a person was no more than having a bundle of characteristics.

It should be remembered that in complex, chaotic systems, whole systems have properties and abilities which cannot be derived from the constituent parts of those systems. When we produce a check list of capabilities that a teacher or doctor or computer programmer must have, we are apt to leave out those higher level characteristics that do not occur in the specified list of capabilities. A 'check list mentality' arises when a person, institution or profession overlooks

* Emoticons are symbols used to express emotions in texts such as emails, e.g. :-) or :-(

those overarching but hard to identify qualities, when the wood cannot be seen for the trees.

So, on the one hand we have the philosophers and educationists who wish to understand learning as a complex process through which a person can become the best they can, and on the other we have politicians and policy makers who, with the help of naïve materialists from the physical and medical sciences, seem determined to analyse education into its smallest components and control it. The irony is that those of us who take a non-material view of education know that the project of the materialists is doomed to failure.

A recognition that knowledge is non-material and socially held led Malcolm to conclude, under the influence of Wittgenstein, that dreams do not have a physical and temporal location the way other mental events do.

If I drive to work, it is possible to say exactly when I saw a traffic light change colour, or observed a pedestrian on a crossing, and where those occurrences took place. But if I dream that I am looking down on my sleeping body, is that dream happening in my head? Or 6 feet above it? Does it happen at some point in the night when I show signs of rapid eye movement? Or does it happen later when I recall it? While there are answers to the set of questions about driving, there is no corresponding set of answers about the dream, because there are no social consequences of answering the question one way or the other. It means that, although we may talk about animals dreaming by way of analogy, we can only really talk about the content of dreams in the case of beings who are in some way able to report them.

This partial lack of connection between mental events and brain events means that the materialist project of 'translating' thoughts into patterns of brain impulses is doomed to failure. As Malcolm argues in the case of dreams, which cannot be directly equated with periods of rapid eye movement sleep, the social reporting of ideas and thoughts is more important than the brain activity that apparently accompanies them.

Thus, from two very different perspectives, both Wittgenstein and Popper argue that the materialist project cannot be successful, and that thoughts are partially autonomous from the brain functions that accompany them.

It would perhaps be appropriate at this point to add a slight gloss to the word 'partial' in the expression 'partial autonomy'. Clearly, mental activity is associated with some brain activity. Neither Popper nor Wittgenstein would wish to argue that thought is possible without a brain. All mental activity is associated with brain activity. What they are denying, however, is that there is a simple, or identifiable correspondence between a particular 'atom' of thought and a particular 'atom' of brain activity, or the firing of specific neurons.

Popper goes further to say that while brain activity will accompany mental activity, the two should not be thought of as happening in parallel. His interest in stressing this point is to argue against what we might consider here a variant of materialism, namely epiphenomenalism. An epiphenomenalist argues that brain activity and mental activity are two facets of the same phenomenon which is only indirectly perceived. As a result, either description is equally valid, but the two accounts refer to something that is essentially 'the same'. The effect of this is to make one of the accounts, normally the account of mental processes, redundant. Popper claims that his previous argument, for the partial autonomy of the contents of thought, is as forceful in demolishing this argument as it was in the case of materialism. Popper argues for an interactionist model, in which thoughts can have an effect upon brain processes and vice versa, without either of them determining the other.

Finally, it is worth considering the perspective of a theorist who might be expected to be more rigorously materialist in his approach. Vygotsky worked under the influence of Marxist science, and was a dialectical materialist, which means that he started from a materialist position.

Vygotsky, as a pupil of Pavlov, argued that the basic or lower mental functions derive from reflexes that we are born with. A newborn baby will turn his or her attention to a loud noise, will suck anything put into his or her mouth, and will curl his or her foot when the sole is tickled. These are fairly basic, physical responses to physical stimuli, and the neural pathways which are associated with them are both simple and relatively easy to identify.

When exposed to social interactions, however, babies are able to re-programme their responses, or transfer them to conditioned stimuli, as when sucking becomes associated with feeding and the satisfaction of hunger, or the response to loud noises becomes attached to a mother's voice, or the calling of the baby's name. Gradually, the baby starts to incorporate socially conditioned responses into its mental repertoire.

Thus, while Vygotsky has a materialist starting point, and retains a materialist view of the lower mental functions, as soon as we come to higher mental functions we are dealing, according to Vygotsky, not with natural or physical brains, but with brains that have in some way been furnished with social and external tools and criteria.

Thus, if I see Arabic numerals (by which I mean numerals as currently used in Arab speaking countries) ۰۱۲۳۴۵۶۷۸۹, I do not immediately associate them with a specific number. I can with relatively little difficulty transpose them to the numerals that I am familiar with. (۱ = 1, ۲ = 2, ۳ = 3, etc.) But they are not, at this moment, part of my mental furniture. Presumably, the numerals that I am so familiar with, and about which I do not even have to think, were once as unfamiliar to me as those that I regard as alien, but I have incorporated then into my thinking to such an extent that I cannot now imagine being without them.

I might once have had to count the symbols on a playing card to know what the meaning of the numeral was, but that was at a time long past. Numbers have become part of my way of thinking to such an extent that they appear to be natural to me.

And so, Vygotsky argues, it is with all our mental functions. They start off as external, social tools and symbols. We are presented with them by parents, friends and teachers. And eventually we incorporate them into our own way of thinking.

The parallels with Popper's argument are striking. For higher mental functions, what is important is that they have social application before they are associated with any brain function of mine. How they are embodied in the brain is unimportant compared to their social and interpersonal validity.

The consequence of this, however, is that we rarely, if ever, encounter a person in their 'natural' state, before they have started to develop their mind by adding in social and cultural symbols and ways of thinking.

According to Vygotsky, the project of education is one of developing self-management, or as he described it 'mastery', by adding cultural ways of thinking to our natural ways of thinking. Thus, we internalize processes which we have first encountered in our relationships with other people, and develop ever improved ways of thinking. In this way we have a brain which is infinitely superior to the brain of individuals who lived 2,000 years ago, even though it may not significantly differ from theirs in its basic patterns of neural connections. Our brains incorporate calculus, psychology, modern science, technology, the internet and Google, and theirs did not. These cultural developments are added to our ways of thinking through childhood and into adulthood in developing ways of thinking. We internalize these processes that we see modelled in our surroundings, or in Vygotsky's own words, 'In general, we could say that the relations between higher mental functions were at one time real relations between people' (Rieber, 1997: 103).

'Is a new born baby a self? Yes and no. It feels: it is capable of feeling pain and pleasure. But it is not yet a person in the sense of Kant's two statements: "A person is a subject that is responsible for its actions", and "A person is something that is conscious, at different times, of the numerical identity of its self". Thus a baby is a body – a developing human body – before it becomes a person, a unity of body and mind' (Popper and Eccles, 1983: 115). While this sentiment seems very much in line with the sentiment of Vygotsky, that a person develops his higher mental functions over time and through interaction with others, these are not, in fact the words of Vygotsky, but the words of Karl Popper.

Thus I think that we can see something like a consensual, considered view of the development of the individual, and of education as a process which is primarily directed towards self-understanding, self-management and the development of improved and improving mental capabilities. While actual education frequently falls short of this, and while it seems to be increasingly common to speak of education as a delivery process, education as self-development and self-management is sometimes achieved in the best systems. The shame is that it so rarely forms the central focus of education.

However, I think that we might go further in describing how the brain and mind operate together, and how learning occurs. We are helped in this process by the models that are available to us from chaos theory, or as I would prefer to describe it, complexity theory.

In this context, a complex system is one in which there are multiple feedback loops, so that through adding processes of negative and positive feedback, non-linear responses occur, where very small changes in the initial conditions can lead to very great differences in the outcomes. This effect, known as the butterfly effect, is common in such complex systems as weather formations and the behaviour of large groups.

Complex systems also show other characteristic behaviours, including emergent properties and recursive symmetries. Emergent properties arise because higher levels cannot be reduced, through a process of analysis, simply to what is happening at lower levels. The recognition of a face may involve the recognition of other features, and in turn may rely on recognition of simpler patterns and shapes, but its recognition as a face transcends those components and becomes something else, a new level of understanding. This new level of activity is an emergent property. Recursive symmetries recognize that, because of emergence, what we see at one level in a complex system cannot be equated with what we see at a higher or lower level, but that similar patterns may nevertheless appear at different levels.

Popper and Eccles (1983) suggest that in the brain we are observing a complex system. The brain is composed of different levels of activity, and different modules that interact at different levels. Thus, those parts of the brain that are most directly related to receiving external stimuli seem to be dedicated to a specific purpose, and to respond in very predictable ways to those stimuli. When we see a symbol or hear a sound, particular areas of the brain become active. In that activity, some of the modular components apply positive feedback to stimulate a larger signal, while others apply negative feedback to damp out the signals.

Yet this by no means accounts for all the activity in the brain. There appear to be other areas of the brain whose function it is to integrate and organize the operation of activity at that lowest level. In this way, I am not consciously aware of sensations at particular points of the skin on my legs, or of issuing individual instructions to the innumerable muscles involved; I simply decide to go for a walk, and the lower level functions are managed at a subconscious level (in normal activity).

And it appears that those higher level functions are in turn monitored by yet other parts of the brain, the top-most level being responsible for my consciousness of myself, or self-consciousness. These levels can pass instructions to other levels, so that I can concentrate on hearing a particular noise, or try to remember a particular telephone number.

We can therefore, helpfully, think of the brain as a complex system that has various levels of activity and multiple feedback loops.

At the same time, we may think of the mind in a similar and separate way. Initial reflex responses are modified by the addition of conditioned stimuli. These conditioned stimuli can be further refined, controlled by the addition of language, managed through moral, scientific or other principles encoded in language, and so the processes of the mind become increasingly complex, with accreted layers of feedback.

When I was a toddler, if I was tired and frustrated, I could simply throw myself on the floor and scream and kick, and generally throw a tantrum. Today, much as I would like to do the same on occasion, I have to reflect on how this would appear to other people, which kinds of standards those people would apply, what I have learned about expectations that an adult should be able to manage their emotions to a great extent (though not, of course, perfectly), not to mention the future implications arising from the probable court case or admission to hospital.

The mind, too, is a complex system with multiple feedback loops, and levels that run all the way from my personal feelings to the system of government that I live within. In that sense I never now meet a stranger completely from scratch. We both bring to our first meeting expectations about how a person who looks like this might be expected to behave, and which kinds of responses would be appropriate.

And as noted before, while these two complex systems, the brain and the mind, are in some ways related, and in some ways influence each other, that influence is not one of direct control or of identity. The mind and the brain follow different rules. The brain responds in its own particular way to electrical and chemical stimuli, from outside, and from other parts of itself. The mind responds to other kinds of values and standards; values of logic, of plausibility, of ethics and desirability and so on. And, of course, drugs can only have a direct effect upon the brain, not upon the mind.

This construction, of the brain and mind as two separate, but interacting, complex systems, may seem unnecessarily complicated. But complexity theory solves some problems that arise in the context of normal mechanics. Popper appears to have been greatly exercised over the question of whether the possibility of the mind influencing the brain could lead to transgressions of the first and second laws of thermodynamics. The first law of thermodynamics is the law of conservation of energy, and embodies the idea that energy cannot be created or destroyed, or you cannot get something for nothing. The second law of thermodynamics deals with the tendency of processes to generate lost heat or increased disorder, measured by a growth in entropy. Having satisfied himself that the second law would not be flouted, Popper then examined in some detail the question of the first law.

For my part, I am not sure how important this is. The question arises from the issue of getting something for nothing, and the idea that the mental process or idea should not be able to initiate a physical process.

Popper argues, I think correctly, that this cannot be explained by the quantum uncertainties of modern physics, since thoughts are not random, but follow the purpose and logic of their own construction.

As I say, I am not sure that the question of the first law of thermodynamics is important, as I do not expect that the energy of movement of my car should be supplied by the force of my foot on the accelerator; the petrol provides another source of energy. In that sense, the brain appears to have a constant involvement of energy supplied by respiration, that the thought might need to do no more than steer the outlet of that motion.

Popper seems to be close to that analysis, arguing that: 'I may perhaps mention again that in processes in which World 2 [the world of thought and inner experience] acts upon World 1 [the physical world] we do not need to assume any more than that the physical magnitudes involved are as small as you like – that is, vanishingly small . . . thus they may possibly be below any measurement' (Popper and Eccles, 1983: 545). But this maps directly onto the notion of complex systems and the butterfly effect. Large outcomes, paradigmatically a hurricane in Texas, may be the result of vanishingly small variations, paradigmatically the flap of a butterfly's wing in Brazil that gives its name to the effect. And this is not simply the theoretical outcome of very small variations, but of variations that are in principle below the level of measurement.

The consensus that is to be found among educationists, therefore, regards people as complex systems that are capable of being changed and developed through a process of engaging with their experience. In contrast with this, materialists are seeking a simple schema, a one-to-one mapping of mental processes onto brain processes. Moreover, they expect that they will be able to describe a brain which retains constant, simple processes over a lifetime.

Again, I want to stress that this picture I am drawing of the proponents of brain science as seeking simple, materialistic, even mechanical answers is not, as it might appear, a distorted caricature. Much as I might like to exaggerate the hubris of brain scientists for effect, it would be extremely difficult to present their ambitions in more grandiose terms than they do themselves. Take, for example, a story reported in *The New Scientist* (Huang, 2008). This reported that brain scientists were now on the verge of a major breakthrough that would produce 'a powerful, concise, mathematical law that encapsulates how the brain works' (Huang, 2008: 31) – a sort of neurophysiological equivalent of $E = mc^2$. It turns out, however, that this new law is a version of the 'Bayesian brain' that has been developed by a scientist called Karl Friston. This is an idea that has been around for more than 20 years. And some experts 'say it is hard to know whether Friston's results are ground-breaking or just repackaged old concepts' (Huang, 2008: 32).

In order to examine this, perhaps it is worth looking at the notion of the Bayesian brain more critically. Bayesian statistics has its origins in an entirely different problem, namely the question of how we come to know things, or the philosophy of scientific method.

Bayesian statistics offer a solution to this problem – we estimate the probability of a future event on the basis of our current knowledge. Then we collect more information, by observing whether our initial prediction was true. In that process we arrive at better, meaning more probable, predictions, and repeat the cycle. In this way we are presumed to follow this process, gradually approaching certainty. Such an approach is a justification for the idea that we learn through a process of developing habits of mind; if something works once, it is more likely to work on the following occasion.

There are problems with Bayesian statistics, the most obvious of which is that even after long periods of study we can discover that we were completely wrong. Or, to put this another way, we often maintain habits which turn out to be unproductive. Conversely, we appear, on happy occasions, to be able to learn something important without any need for repetition. So Bayesian statistics appears to be deficient in a number of ways; it does not seem to hold together philosophically, and it does not appear to capture what we actually do when we learn something new. In consequence of this, it has been attacked very vigorously by Popper, who argued that Bayesian statistics was simply a sophisticated restatement of the principle of scientific induction.

It is not absolutely necessary to come to a conclusion on this question, although I certainly prefer Popper's arguments on this question. What is crucial, however, is to note that this so-called 'breakthrough' depends upon the application of a theory which is hotly contested. It is not quite as straightforward as it appears at first glance.

There are two aspects of the critique of Bayesian statistics which are crucial in the context of learning. In the first place, it appears that we can, and often do, learn from a single, critical event. In addition, it does not seem that moving from one position to another of greater probability is necessarily a positive move; risk taking and the development of new lines of thought are crucial to long term advance.

What Friston adds to the standard model of the Bayesian brain is the concept of free energy, using this to describe the supposed brain mechanism of removing error by incorporating new information into the brain's estimates or predictions. Whether free energy is actually being proposed as a mechanism that explains this supposed tendency to reduce error, or whether the notion of free energy is simply another way of describing the process, is not clear, and leaves room for the doubt as to whether Friston's ideas are new or are old ones repackaged. It is the difference between a model which may be helpful in explaining how the brain works and a supposed account of how it does work. As I have noted elsewhere (Turner, 2007: 21) scientists are not necessarily as careful as they should be in distinguishing between these two.

But what this illustrates is that, even in *The New Scientist*, which is by no means as cavalier with its presentation of science as some parts of the popular press, a materialistic, mechanical interpretation of mental functions can be put forward as though it were part of a consensus. This makes it easier to understand why many of those only peripherally engaged with education would adopt simplistic and materialistic interpretations of educational processes.

Of greater concern are those approaches which seem to be gaining increased ground among educators, which base their arguments on the supposed findings of brain-science. A range of techniques which include the word 'brain' have been advanced as the new way forward to improve education. Brain training, brain-based education and so on are very much in vogue. So it would be appropriate to focus on some aspects of these approaches. I will focus, for the sake of this discussion, on the book *Brain-Based Learning* by Eric Jensen. In many ways this is a book which makes modest claims, and tries to deal with the evidence in a most responsible way. Even so, the sub-title of the book still proclaims it to be the 'new paradigm of teaching' – the book is not without ambition in relation to changing how we teach.

The book is set out in chapters, each of which aims to introduce an aspect of our understanding of the functioning of the brain, to develop this understanding to identify the implications for learning, and conclude with recommendations as to how a classroom teacher should structure his/her activities as a result. Because each chapter follows this complex trajectory, it is worth looking at the arguments in some detail. After all, if the book is successful it represents a major step forward in terms of a materialistic understanding of brain function.

By way of illustration, I shall start by examining the third chapter of the book, 'Brain dominance in learning'. This addresses the question which has been raised already, that certain mental functions can be located in one hemisphere of the brain.

The first point to note is that Jensen is by no means sensationalist in the presentation of evidence regarding lateral division in the brain.

> Old myths die hard. Much of the original work of Nobel Laureate Roger Sperry, who discovered the functioning differences between left and right hemisphere of the brain remains valid today. But the spin put on his research also remains. Forty years after his discovery, we still hear people talk of 'left-brained people' and 'right-brained people', which is not just anatomically incorrect (unless one has a hemispherectomy), but can also be pejorative labeling . . . The prevailing research in neuroscience avoids the definitive left-versus-right labels. Scientists now use the term relative lateralization: the brain is designed to process spatially from left to right hemisphere, but it processes time (past to future) from back to front. In short, on any given day, you'll use most of your brain, most of the time . . . It is an oversimplification to say that an individual is left-brained or right-brained. We are all whole-brained (but see Figure 3.1 for a list of attributes that are characteristic of each hemisphere). (Jensen, 2008: 19)

The language here is interesting. Jensen describes the most radical aspects of brain lateralization as 'a myth' – a myth that has been dispelled in very much those terms by both the TLRP (2007) and the OECD (2007). So what is clear here is that Jensen is presenting the actual state of knowledge in brain science in a careful way. The evidence for laterality is derived from patients suffering from such a radical, and literal, separation of the hemispheres that it is doubtful whether the experiments tell us much of value about normal subjects, those who have not had a hemispherectomy.

But in a move that is very reminiscent of promissory materialism, Jensen manages in a single sentence to assert that we are whole brained, and that, nevertheless, there is a relative dominance of hemispheres in relation to particular mental capacities.

> Figure 3.1 lists the following characteristics of left-brain and right-brain dominant learners:
>
> Left-brain-dominant learners, more often than not, may
> - Prefer things in sequence
> - Learn best from parts to wholes
> - Prefer a phonetic reading system
> - Like words, symbols, and letters
> - Rather read about a subject first
> - Want to gather related factual information
> - Prefer detailed orderly instructions
> - Experience more internal focus
> - Want structure and predictability.
>
> Right-brain-dominant learners, more often than not, may
> - Be more comfortable with randomness
> - Learn best from wholes to parts
> - Prefer a whole-language reading system
> - Like pictures, graphs, and charts
> - Rather see or experience a subject first
> - Want to gather information about relationships among things
> - Prefer spontaneous, go-with-the-flow, learning environments
> - Experience more external focus
> - Want open-ended approaches, novelty, and surprises.

Source: (Used with permission of Corwin Press: from Eric Jensen, 2008 (2nd Edition) *Brain-based Learning*, page 20; permission conveyed through Copyright Clearance Center, Inc.)

The chapter continues with accounts of PET scans and EEG scans. These report the facts about the way certain parts of the brain seem to be activated in certain mental operations, but this is a measured presentation, and by no means dogmatic.

The chapter concludes with a final box, entitled, 'What this means to you', which makes the following practical suggestion for teachers in the classroom:

> Provide learners with global overviews as well as step-by-step instructions. Represent the learning plan depicting the big picture, followed by details representing the subtopics. Alternate between the big picture and the details. (Jensen, 2008: 22)

What is remarkable about this is that the advice to alternate between the big picture and the details, which may indeed be very sound advice, has no discernible connection with the claim that the big picture is processed in the right brain and details are processed in the left brain. Its strength, if it has a strength, stands or falls on the basis of classroom experience. Alternating between big picture and detail simultaneously caters for individual differences, catering for those who prefer to receive the big picture first and for those who prefer to get the details first, and it also caters for the different aspects of each individual's understanding, and the eventual need to understand different levels of the topic being studied. And my own classroom experience, anecdotal though it is, disposes me to believe that it is good advice.

But, and this point is crucial, it would still be good advice if the big picture was processed in the toes and the details were processed in the ear lobes. Or, indeed, if specific mental functions could not be localized at all.

The brain science which is called upon to support the teaching method, which, in fact, is claimed to be the basis of the 'new paradigm of teaching' is more or less completely irrelevant to the teaching guidance offered. Aside from the obvious damage which this does to the value that we attach to the logical construction of arguments, this book seems harmless enough. It advocates benign approaches to teaching, and it reports responsibly what the current state of brain science is. Unfortunately it asserts a link between those two functions which is completely unsupported.

A recent paper published in the *Journal of Cognitive Neuroscience*, entitled 'The Seductive Nature of Neuroscience Explanations', tested people's evaluations of explanations that purported to account for functions of the mind (Weisberg et al., 2008: 471–2). The authors found that people found explanations that included reference to neuroscience language and results were more highly regarded than those that did not, even when the content of the neuroscience added nothing substantive to the explanation. (To their credit, this effect was not found among neuroscientists, although it was even more marked in students of neuroscience than it was in the general public.) We perhaps need to be aware of this seductive nature of neuroscientific explanations when we read accounts that claim to design educational measures based on brain science, or when trying to understand how such accounts have such a strong appeal for the general public.

Let me stress again that, on the whole, I find the practical suggestions that Jensen offers measured and likely to promote good practice in the classroom. In some cases I would go further and say that I thoroughly applaud his conclusions. To take another example, Chapter 15 deals with motivation and rewards. Somewhat surprisingly, it seems to me, Jensen concludes that extrinsic motivation has a negative effect on learning, and in the long run is detrimental to the personal development of the learner. I say 'somewhat surprisingly' because this advice is diametrically opposed to the advice normally given in systems of behaviour management for teachers. On the other hand, it is strongly reminiscent of the argument that I put forward in relation to intrinsic and extrinsic motivation in a different context (Postman, 1985).

However, Jensen buttresses his argument with a statement of the 'essential understanding' in the field of motivation:

> The essential understanding here is that we are all biologically driven to seek out new learning. The human brain loves to learn; our very survival, in fact, is dependent on learning. Usually our motivation looks as if it is the pursuit of curiosity, novelty, social contact, food sources, shelter, and enjoyment. Learners have a built-in motivation that does not require a teacher's input or manipulation to work. Our brains have hungrily absorbed information, integrated it, made meaning out of it, remembered it, and used it at appropriate times for eons. At school, if we use our natural motivations and curiosity, we can expect students to learn better and enjoy more. (Jensen, 2008: 119)

I am really not sure that curiosity is a biological drive, or what is gained by stressing the naturalness, or evolutionary advantage, of learning.

Jensen supports his argument with a diagram of the brain, pinpointing the location of the thalamus, and the production of dopamine. In a curiously structured discussion, Jensen suggests that external rewards (or as he would say bribes) follow a law of diminishing returns. He develops this with the parallel that the body becomes habituated to a drug such as cocaine, and that the effectiveness of external rewards diminishes with use. For reasons which, I am afraid, are beyond me, he concludes that we should therefore rely on a different drug system, that of dopamine.

Let me say again, I agree very strongly with the conclusions that Jensen comes to.

> Consider, for example, a school that is having problems with truancy and low attendance. The administrative staff decides, as an incentive, to reward those who come every day. Now each student gets a reward for having 100 percent attendance during the month . . . Students immediately feel bribed for coming to school. They think, 'The situation must be really bad for them to bribe us.' But learners still respond to the rewarded behaviour. 'It's stupid, but we'll play the game', they say. Now school is about working the system instead of learning. (Jensen, 2008: 122)

I am fully persuaded by that argument, and I believe that it has been put forward elegantly and logically. But I cannot see what is added by discussion of the thalamus and dopamine. Extrinsic motivation is risky, whatever happens or does not happen in the brain.

Going through the book *Brain-Based Learning* (Jensen, 2008), this pattern is repeated again and again. Similar examples could be given in relation to the many different varieties of brain-based education or brain training.

However, although it happens that I agree with most of Jensen's specific recommendations for classroom management, there is no reason to suppose that all recommendations derived from brain science would be compatible with those derived by Jensen, or preferred by me.

Since, as I have argued, there is little or no connection between the exposition of brain science and suggestions for teachers, reference to neurophysiology can be claimed as support for almost anything at all, in much the same way as, in formal logic, any statement can be derived from a contradiction.

It is difficult to say whether this line of argument might be the outcome of a cynical attempt on the part of authors to advance promissory materialism, or a pragmatic acceptance of the fact that many teachers seem to find reference to brain science convincing, and that one might as well use that weakness of teachers to make sure some positive methods are adopted. However, my fear is that, in much the same way that extrinsic motivation damages intrinsic motivation, use of poor arguments undermines the strength of good arguments. For that reason I am arguing here that it is important to make clear the very weak links between brain science and classroom conduct.

As educators and as educationists, we need the courage to make plain that the ultimate test of educational recommendations, apart from their internal logic, is whether they work in the classroom. Whatever lights up, or does not light up, in a PET scan, the acid test for a recommendation to teachers is whether it has positive educational effects in the classroom, and the strength of educational evidence outweighs any amount of psychological or neuropsychological demonstration.

Throughout this exploration of the issues relating to the relationship between the brain and the mind I have stressed that there are two approaches – a simplistic, scientific approach and a philosophical approach which engages the complexity of the actual situation. There is, however, a possible compromise, namely a scientific approach which embraces complexity. Such an approach is available to us in the form of complexity theory, or chaos theory as it is sometimes called.

The traditional approach employed in science is an analytical, or atomistic, one. The basic assumption is that complex phenomena can be broken down into their constituent building blocks, or atoms, and that once all of the atoms have been understood, they can be reassembled to produce an understanding of the whole.

Although I have described this approach as scientific, atomism has been much more widespread than that. It has also been a strong influence in some philosophical approaches. In the context of understanding the workings of the mind, we have seen atomism employed to understand both the workings of the brain, and the working of the mind.

This atomism is at the heart of the project of promissory materialism. It breaks down the functions of the brain into the firing of neurons, and it breaks down the functions of the mind into such simple activities as laying down memory or recalling an item previously stored, or of atomic elements of perception. The final stage of this project involves the connecting together of the atoms of brain function with the atoms of thought. If this project was achievable, the step from a dancing worm to the control of thought would be a simple and logical one.

The alternative insights offered by chaos theory can also be derived from aspects of a scientific approach, but the relationship between atoms and larger structures is quite different.

Chaos theory deals with the science of such phenomena as weather patterns, compound pendulums and various other systems. I have discussed elsewhere the possible application of complexity theory to educational phenomena (Turner, 2007).

Importantly, chaotic systems are those which involve multiple feedback loops, which give rise to the possibility that very small changes in state can produce very large differences in outcomes (the so-called butterfly effect). In addition, complex systems demonstrate recursive symmetry, in which patterns at lower levels are repeated at higher levels, and emergent properties, or properties that are evident at higher levels but cannot be reduced to the sum of phenomena at lower levels.

Some indication of the import of these features can be given by considering the workings of a computer, which does not exhibit them. Thus, if we wish a computer to remember a number (which is all that a computer can remember) we have to instruct it what the number is, and, equally importantly, where to save it. (Obviously, as a mere typist, I do not actually have to decide, letter by letter, where the computer is going to save each letter that I type, either in the long run or the short run. Most of this process is handled automatically by the software that I am using, and I only have to remember the more gross descriptions that I give to the data, such as the name of the file.) Conversely, if I want the computer to retrieve a number for a particular purpose, I have to tell it where to find that number.

In that very simple system lie huge possibilities for mistakes. The computer cannot possibly know whether the number that it retrieves when it goes to the address that it has been given is appropriate for the purpose that it is going to be put to. If it finds the number, it has to assume that it is correct.

What happens when I retrieve some data from memory, however, is quite different, as we can clearly see if we consider those occasions when we have to work hard to retrieve the memory.

I am trying, for example, to remember the name of an actor or actress, which just escapes me. I might be able to remember one or more roles they played in different films. (I might not be able to remember exactly the titles of the films, but I might remember the circumstances in which I saw them.) I may associate those films with certain sights, sounds and smells, and with specific emotional responses, which might or might not be attached to the film, or to the people that I saw the film with, or with events connected with the film.

I can remember, for example, that I saw the film *Bullitt*, with Steve McQueen, in 1970, because the film includes a famous car chase sequence, which had a particularly strong emotional effect on me because I went to see the film a week after I had had a very serious car accident while driving my mother's car.

Saving and retrieving memory, therefore, are not, as they are in the case of a computer, a simple system that involves placing one piece of data into one place and keeping hold of the address. Human memory is a whole range of memory processes that link several associated memories, not only the fact of the matter to be remembered, but details of how we learned it and other associated circumstances. In each of these memory paths there are branching cross connections and feedback, so that if we cannot remember the name of the actor or actress, we can try to reconstruct the memory from the clues that we can retrieve. We might even be able to make these hints explicit, and try to get somebody else to help us remember the name. When eventually we do remember, or somebody else suggests a name to us, we know instantly whether it is right or not, because all of the pieces 'come together' to make an intelligible whole.

Thus it makes sense to say of a person that he or she is trying to remember something. It makes no sense at all to say that a computer is trying to remember something. In the case of the computer, the programme is given an address where it can find a stored piece of data. It goes to the address and retrieves the data, which can be right or wrong, appropriate or inappropriate, but it cannot be half remembered, or only recovered by extended effort.

At the heart of human memory, and all human thought, is the process of making sense. Making sense is not a simple process, but is a complex process in which several, possibly many, parallel processes coincide. A sentence makes sense because the meaning of the words that compose it and the grammar and syntax of the sentence fit together. But we also compare the meaning with the context, with our memory, our understanding of the character of the person who spoke it, our wishes and feelings. All of these come together for us to tell us whether the utterance makes sense, or whether there is something here that we need more information on.

Making sense, or comprehensibility, is a complex, emergent property. We are aware of occasions when we understood all the words that were spoken, but had no idea of what was being said. Comprehension cannot be broken down into its constituent atoms in that way. Mental processes and understanding are gestalt phenomena, holistic phenomena, which cannot be subjected to an atomistic approach.

Similarly, brain function is a complex phenomenon that cannot be understood as the sum of the activity of individual neurons.

Brain and mind, therefore, match in the sense that they are both complex and chaotic systems which cannot be reduced to the activities of their component parts. And doubtless we will, in time, learn more about how they work together. But we will never be able to find a direct correspondence between the functioning of the two, because in both the butterfly effect is at work, where very tiny differences have a huge effect on the outcome.

A standard, atomistic approach, the traditional approach of science, has looked at sequences of causation. Each event follows on, one after the other, like links in a chain. Mental processes, and we must suppose brain processes, do not work in that way.

While working away at this chapter, the phone rings. A student is on the line, who wishes to discuss with me a piece of work that she has sent me. I turn my thoughts from what I had been thinking about with full concentration only a fraction of a second earlier, and try to remember what I can of the piece of work that I have read. She elaborates her themes, corrects my memory on a few points, and we agree a time and date to meet and discuss it more fully in the following week. I put the date in my diary, finish the telephone conversation, and hang up.

I take a few minutes reading over my last notes to work out what I was thinking about before the telephone call. And before long I am back in the train of thought that is where I was before, as though the telephone call had never happened. And, unless I have been visited by the man from Porlock, most interruptions will happen in this way, occurring but leaving very little trace on the processes on which they have intruded.

However, roughly a week later a glance at my diary will remind me of the agreement to meet, and I will go to the meeting to continue the conversation that was started in the telephone conversation.

In this way, human experience is typically not a single chain of events one causing the other, but intersecting and interrupting chains of events that 'cause' one another, and which are driven, each by its own internal logic or comprehensibility. I put 'cause' in quotes in this latter case, because it is clearly not the same meaning of the word that we normally employ where a complete chain of events links through from beginning to end.

But in this case, it is not the reading of ink marks in a book that makes me set off for a meeting. It is the fact that the words have meaning, not only in terms of what they say, or in terms of the fact that they are in my diary, or indeed that I can remember putting them into my diary. All of those things come together to create a meaning, and an understanding of the intention that I had when I put the date in my diary, even though I can see no obvious material link between one event and the other.

What people have in common is a very strong, possibly irresistible, drive to make sense out of their experience. This means that meaning is the most important aspect of mental experience, but that meaning is least capable of being captured in a simple, an atomistic or a materialist framework. Vygotsky has noted that psychology which depends upon a simple stimulus response pattern is capable only of capturing those aspects of human endeavour which are closest to animals (Reiber, 1997: 37).

That is to say, lower mental functions may be described and accounted for in terms of the material functions of the brain. If I hit my thumb with a hammer I may shout out and scream in pain. The outburst might be accounted for in terms of a response to pain. What I shout will be shaped by previous experience, cultural values, who is in earshot, who I think is in earshot, and a host of other considerations which have an impact that cannot easily be described.

In this sense, speech is unlike any other activity. Not only is the meaning important and not aligned directly with any specific physical condition, but I hear what I say and there is immediate feedback as my own speech forms part of the input to my next thought.

This basic feature of speech, which is also a feature of thought, makes the sequence of thoughts ineffable.

Put in that light we can see how obsessed our society has become with a materialist approach to understanding our being. We believe that a person cannot understand him- or herself without being able to know his or her genetic parents, and possibly being able to trace his or her origins through many generations. We believe that genetics have an important, even dominant, role in defining our potential.

If we wish education to develop in a better way we need to address directly the central problem, namely that those who design our educational system, indeed many of those who take part in our educational system, do not really understand how it works. They believe that learning is a material process, when it is not. It is going to be hard work to persuade people that education is a process through which people acquire self-management; indeed, if we put it in Popper's terms, it is the process by which physical bodies become a 'self'. Above all, if education is about learners developing self-management, the most important first step is that learners should understand that to be the case.

But perhaps equally importantly, we need to overturn the materialistic understanding which is widely held, including by those who have political responsibility for regulating the state system of education. Morris (2008: 9), a former Secretary of State for education in the UK, suggests that when politicians face a decision, and the evidence contradicts their instincts or common sense, they are more likely to rely upon their instincts. The very fact that she presents the idea that a political choice might be a matter of instinct gives a hint that a materialistic viewpoint lurks in her formulation of political and educational processes:

> And sometimes politicians have this battle between what the evidence tells them and what their political instincts tell them and on most occasions they'll back their political instincts more than they will the evidence; that's the nature of being a politician. (Morris, 2008: 9)

Although Morris goes on to note that this is specific to education, in the sense that in the area of health politicians are unlikely to get involved in the same level of detail, it is important to understand exactly what those instincts are. And this is especially true because, as I have noted, everybody believes that they know about education, and reliance on common sense, outdated practices or personal anecdotes is rife.

Introducing an educational system which focuses on changing people for the better and developing self-management is extremely important. Society has moved on from a time when people could be forced to learn because those in authority said so. Teachers feel this loss of authority particularly keenly. But there is no going back. Nor is there any going back to the days when those who could not be forced into education could be expelled from it. Nowadays, everybody must be educated in order that they can survive in today's complex society.

The way forward is to embrace the idea of an education for self-management and self-development, and engage learners as active partners in designing their own education. But this will not be possible so long as a wider public thinks of education in material terms, as something that is done to them, as skills and knowledge (or worse still, certificates) that they acquire on their passage through school.

In this context, we can see how damaging demands for more and more externally imposed discipline are. They defer, postpone or abort the real project, which is the development of self-discipline.

And at the same time we need to be educating everybody else who has a stake in education.

Chapter 11

Conclusions

Overall, I have used the idea of 'smart drugs', medication that can enhance mental function, as a way of examining our assumptions about intelligence, learning and education in general. The most important finding was the very strong influence that promissory materialism has on thinking in this area. Even where authors are quite critical of a simplistic use of brain science, and even when they deliberately set out to dispel false ideas arising from neuroscience, they seem to find it impossible to relinquish the hope that in some unspecified future, near or far, brain science will provide all the answers that we need to understand education and learning. The idea that we are calculating machines and that biology is on the verge of providing us with the instruction manual dies very hard.

In contrast with this, the long history of brain science has been more notable for its failures than for its successes. With the benefit of hindsight, and some distance, we can now see that phrenology was a misleading diversion from the road to understanding human development. What is less clear is whether we have really learned the lesson, or whether we are in danger of repeating similar mistakes with greater technical efficiency.

The most sceptical voice is that of Bruer (1997), who argued that the idea that brain science could inform education was 'a bridge too far'. But the implication of this is that the connection between brain science and psychology, and between psychology and education, are not bridges too far. Psychology will one day be explained in terms of brain science, which is exactly the promise of promissory materialism.

That particular link is not central to my concerns. I do not believe that psychology can be seen as capable of reduction to a materialist base, but if it can, that is simply another indication of the weakness of psychology. Vygotsky argued that one of the reasons why psychology was so poor in explanatory power was because psychologists restricted themselves to a single, simple mechanism, mainly that of stimulus and response. He also argued that one consequence of that failing is that psychology is much more effective when dealing with lower mental functions – functions that are the most basic, instinctive and animal in us – than in dealing with higher mental functions. In short, if the bridge between brain science and psychology is sound, it is because it links to the least interesting parts of psychology.

I certainly do not wish to deny that there are more interesting parts to psychology, particularly in more recent developments in social psychology. But if psychology could be reduced to neuroscience, that would be because it was a very poor psychology indeed.

Looking at the second bridge, from psychology to education, that is a bridge that is of more concern to me, but it seems no more secure than the first. Education is not a process that is concerned exclusively with what happens in the consciousness of a single individual. Vygotsky reminds us that all higher mental functions start out as relationships between people. Learning and development depend upon social interaction and social context. Learning is not about the content of a single, isolated mind, much less about the connections of a single, isolated brain.

It is also worth noting that, from a very different perspective, Popper argued that our knowledge has an existence that is in some ways independent of our knowing it. Statements can be true or false, quite independently of how strongly we believe in them or how repugnant we find them. Different pieces of knowledge, and the implications of different assumptions, interact and have consequences quite independently of our convenience. Knowledge is not the sum total of what is held in our brains; it is something else beyond that. Consequently, learning cannot be a process of establishing the right connections between our neurons.

Yet we find it very easy to talk as though it was our brain that needed educating rather than us. We are certainly comfortable about book titles such as *The Brain's Behind It*, or *The Learning Brain*. And, thanks to Nintendo, the expression 'brain training' and the idea that a young brain is better than an old one, seem to be entering the popular consciousness. We even see organizations, such as the International Brain Education Association, dedicated to spreading the word that what we need is better educated brains.

It is, of course, obvious, but nevertheless needs to be stressed, that brains do not exist in isolation. We learn and develop in social contexts, and what we understand is shaped by the way in which we learn it and the people who help us to learn. For this reason, education and an understanding of learning can never be reduced to psychology.

For the opposite reasons, education can never be reduced to sociology either. Learning and education is not only or exclusively about the social, but also involves the internal, the mental process, and in particular the self-management of those mental processes. Education stands at the cusp between the personal and the social and cannot be properly understood if either of those aspects is omitted.

Again, the way in which Vygotsky explained learning, as involving first an interpersonal cycle in which the individual can be helped and supported in a task, followed by an intrapersonal cycle in which the person has to decide for him- or herself how to incorporate the learning of the first cycle into their personal frameworks for understanding, is helpful. Indeed, in performing this intrapersonal cycle, the person is developing their own person, providing the terms of reference within which they will exercise self-discipline.

This is not a negative comment, or a suggestion that education is too difficult to understand. On the contrary, it suggests that education is a good and positive focus for social science research, as any problem that might arise in other areas of study must arise even more severely in education. This suggests that developing a better understanding of education may help in the development of other, and better, social sciences.

But having come this far, what stands out is the extent to which the contrary opinion dominates education policy and public pronouncements on education. The idea that medical models are appropriate for educational settings is at the heart of any attempt to medicate ourselves to better ways of thinking. Attention Deficit Hyperactivity Disorder is described as a medical condition which can be appropriately treated with drugs. This ignores entirely the obvious fact that failure to pay attention and an inclination towards restlessness are a perfectly appropriate response on the part of a normal human being to certain social settings. For me, that might be exposure to large amounts of soap operas and reality TV, or a pep talk on the importance of commercial values to academe. For others it might be a professorial lecture or having to read a book on brain science. But in neither case would medication be the appropriate response.

We are in danger of falling too easily into a mindset where learning is seen as being automatically better than not learning, and change is seen as being preferable to lack of change. Worse than that, we are in danger of stating that learning and changing are 'normal' states of affairs, and that failure to learn, or failure to change, is a symptom of some underlying malady or a sign of psychological or emotional weakness or immaturity. Learning and change are characterized as 'challenging', and those who are unable to embrace them need support to overcome their emotional response to that challenge.

This involves a very serious narrowing of what counts as a normal, human response. There are some things that should not be learned, and there are some changes that should be resisted because they are unimportant, irrelevant or simply the reflection of the latest fad. The idea that resistance to learning and change are symptoms of a medical condition is dehumanizing. In order to overcome this very prevalent trend in educational thought, we should, perhaps, seek out exemplars of heroic resistance to learning and/or change. We might start with Nelson Mandela's refusal to learn that it was appropriate to base a society on racial discrimination. We might continue with Johannes Kepler's refusal to learn that planets travel on unpredictable paths. And we might round off with consideration of George Washington's inability to learn that a politician should be economical with the truth. No doubt, that is not the end of the examples, and the reader may have his or her own favourites.

We should therefore be seriously concerned about this approach to education as a physical, medical process. It is widespread – 'Everyone knows you can prevent muscle loss with exercise, and use such activities to improve your body over time. And the same could be said for your brain' (Nintendo, 2006) – but it is mistaken. It is based on the same thinking that leads us to believe that medication can be effective in promoting better thinking. Both are rooted in a simplistic materialism.

However, our concerns should extend beyond the question of whether some questionable classroom practices are gaining in popularity, or whether some charlatans are growing rich from selling an attractive but useless recipe for improvement. The attitudes which make brain training attractive extend into a very wide range of policy questions, not least who is considered an appropriate 'expert' to comment on educational issues.

The radio programme, *The Defeat of Sleep* (BBC, 2007), which first set me off on an exploration of the issues behind smart drugs, included commentary from a range of specialists. These included specialists in sleep disorders, animal psychologists, neuro-pharmacologists, psychologists, medical ethicists and parents. Notable for its absence was any perspective from a specialist in education. Almost by definition, specialists in education are deemed to be non-specialists. It is another strand of promissory materialism that the knowledge held by teachers and educationists is due, shortly, to be overtaken by the knowledge provided by 'hard' scientists, at which point the public will have access to a full understanding of education, and the teachers and specialists in education will be redundant. Nor is it enough that such action should be threatened for the future; in anticipation we already seek the views of other specialists on education ahead of those who actually work in schools and classrooms. We need, therefore, to be extremely wary of always thinking that other specialists, particularly doctors and psychologists, have direct access to some special understanding of educational issues.

These attitudes are multiplied through a process of funding research which itself relies upon expert opinion. You can be fairly sure that any proposed research which addresses questions of learning and teaching will be scrutinized by psychologists, who will be invited to give an opinion as to whether the proposal constitutes good research or not. Those who have most to gain, therefore, from an adherence to promissory materialism, and an acceptance of medical models of development, have a powerful say in where money is invested for future research in education. It is perhaps relevant to compare the British Educational Research Association (BERA) and the British Psychological Association (BPS). In 2007, BERA employed two members of staff, maintained offices in Macclesfield (BERA, 2008) and published two regular journals, while the BPS employed 127 staff, maintained its head office in Leicester and regional offices in Belfast, Cardiff, Glasgow and London (BPS, 2007) and published a dozen journals. Of course, the interests and activities of the BPS are not by any means restricted to educational psychology, but this contrast does highlight rather dramatically the difference in resources which are available in the two fields of endeavour.

There are important dangers here, especially when the pursuit of research funding has become an end in itself, and not merely a means of securing resources for research, that funding will be diverted away from research that is of value for the practice of education and into areas that are of interest mainly to researchers in other fields. This is partly the case in relation to the involvement of psychologists in educational research, as psychologists tend to lean towards medical models of research themselves, and to have little interest in the more difficult areas of classroom research or the messiness of everyday educational settings. But it is, of course, much worse in the case of medical research. All of that work that is being done to use brain scans to identify which parts of the brain are active in which circumstances has to be paid for, and educational research can ill-afford the diversion of money and effort into areas that are of little current interest.

A cynic might suggest that promissory materialism was less of a research strategy, and more of a promissory note designed to transfer research resources from the cash-strapped area of educational research and into the resource-rich area of medical research. But whether that is a deliberate strategy or not, it should hardly be medics and psychologists who have the final word on the transfer of that money.

However, this is not only about conflict between cognate areas of the social sciences. We can see similar struggles fought out over 'big science' and 'little science' in such areas as physics and chemistry. Faced with the need to justify the expenditure of several million pounds of public money on research, government agencies find it easier to contemplate large, high technology projects in preference to a larger number of small projects of lower technical status but of higher social impact. In this way research on nuclear energy wins out over energy conservation measures, research on new drugs treatments appeals more than preventative medicine and large scale urban restructuring looks more attractive than repairing the existing housing stock. The grand gesture appeals to politicians more than solid hard work below the radar of public attention, especially if it involves investment in shiny new technical equipment. The glamour of promissory materialism can be very persuasive.

On the other hand, there is little incentive or appetite for private investment in education, a sphere that is dominated by public institutions. Research into a potential smart drug may lead to the opening up of a market of hundreds of thousands of dollars annually, quite apart form the legitimate use of that drug to treat Parkinson's disease or senile dementia. Few areas of educational research can offer anything like the returns available to pharmaceutical companies. And while there is little scope for private profit to influence investment in educational research, the converse is not the case; government funding is often encouraged to flow into areas where there is private investment. This can result in even less funding of educational research than would otherwise be the case.

The idea that intelligence has a basis that is purely physical, therefore, leads to damage at a number of levels in the education system. The most damaging, because the most widespread, is the fact that it supports the idea, accepted by many individual learners, that they are incapable. As Dweck (1999) has noted, those who believe that intelligence depends upon some physical endowment that they lack, rapidly learn patterns of helplessness. Also at a personal level, although as yet, mercifully, on a less widespread scale, individual interventions to 'treat' learning disorders do untold damage. Rather than learn to accommodate difference, and find a way where a broad range of talent can be recognized, we classify the abnormal as pathological, and set about its treatment.

Not, of course, that we are always logical in our educational prescriptions. At the same time as doing untold damage to the self-esteem of young people, by explaining to them that they are incapable of learning without the support of drugs, we insist that everything possible should be done to boost the self-esteem of all young people. We know, or think that we know, that high self-esteem is a characteristic of capable people, so we therefore conclude, quite wrongly, that if we boost self-esteem we will make people capable. Increasing people's self-esteem will help their performance up to a point, but nowhere near as much as an accurate self-evaluation of their performance. We can all think of (at least a few) people who are brimming with self-esteem, but who are fundamentally incapable in their professional area. If boosting self-esteem is an answer, it is at best a very partial answer, and runs the risk of infantilizing learners by suggesting that they cannot learn without the constant emotional crutch of praise.

But at a broader social and cultural level, promissory materialism can also do considerable damage, by diverting much needed resources away from education and into other areas of research which have not been shown to have any beneficial effect on education at all.

There is the further difficulty that a pseudo-scientific association between mind and brain has the function of legitimizing certain activities over others in an unjustified way. Thus, games that are seen as 'brain training' come to be seen as legitimate, while those that are not come to be seen as 'play' and 'time wasting'. I think that we need to be quite clear about this. I do not, in any way, object to the idea of games being educational, or of learning through play. But adults specialize in turning play into work for children. For example, Froebel structured the education of young children around a series of 'gifts', typically a set of wooden bricks that could be used in imaginative play to build a house, a ship, a shop, a dining room suite, a box of chocolates, in fact anything that a more fertile imagination than mine might like to envisage. But Froebel's followers could not resist adding books of instructions, with blueprints, indicating exactly how the blocks could be used to build a palace, or an ocean liner. Those followers were, presumably, keen to promote efficiency and 'time on task'.

At which point it stops being play and becomes children's work, and children are particularly adept at spotting that particular transition. Education cannot be improved by an efficiency drive and a time and motion study. We all know that we learn best when we are not on task. The richest learning comes when we have prepared ourselves well, but are perhaps not concentrating too intently at the instant – perhaps thinking about something quite different – when suddenly we have an insight that makes everything much clearer. Sleep may also play a role in this process, as when we fall asleep thinking about a problem. We do not, however, learn while we are asleep; we learn when we wake with a new idea to try out, and reflect consciously on the application of that idea. So, for example, I may fall asleep after an extended search for a book, and wake with a new thought about a place where I might look for it. My learning comes from going and checking whether the book is where I dreamt it was, not from my dreaming about the book. Learning is a process of developing self-management through a sequence of personal experiences.

Anything that suggests that learning can be, or should be, an efficient process that is disconnected from experience is likely to have a damaging influence on education at all the levels described above. That would include everything from the notion that we can measure intelligence independently from the experience of the person concerned to the idea that people can learn effectively without reflection, perhaps while unconscious in sleep. But of all of those simplistic, and damaging, approaches to education, the most damaging is that intelligence can be boosted pharmacologically, and that thinking better is about increasing the connections between neurons in the brain.

People are complex, self-regulating systems with multiple feedback loops. This means that it is impossible to predict precisely what anyone will do in particular circumstances. I am not sure what that means for the future of educational research or for the opportunities that are available to improve educational practice. What I am clear about is that thinking of ourselves as any kind of calculating machine is going to impede our progress along that path. And the belief that a pill can be used to make us smarter is a symptom of how little we have understood about how we really do learn.

References

Academy of Medical Sciences (2008) *Brain Science, Addiction and Drugs* (London: Academy of Medical Sciences) available at http://www.acmedsci.ac.uk/download.php/file=_images_project_BrainSci (accessed 23 May 2008).

Baker, S and Brown, B. J. (2007) *Rethinking Universities: The Social Functions of Higher Education* (London: Continuum).

BBC (2007) *The Defeat of Sleep* (London: BBC) broadcast on 16 April 2007. Some details are available at http://www.bbc.co.uk/radio4/science/pip/expdl/ (accessed 27 May 2009).

Bee, Peta (2007) 'Smart Drugs for Straight As' in *The Times*, 14 May 2007, *Times* 2, pp. 8–9.

Belkin, L., Kurtzberg, T. and Naquin, C. (2008) 'Being Honest Online: The Finer Points of Lying in Online Ultimatum Bargaining', a paper presented at the annual meeting of the Academy of Management, 8–13 August, Anaheim, California.

BERA (2008) British Educational Research Association website http://www.bera.ac.uk/index.php (accessed 9 July 2008).

Bernstein, N. A. (1996) *On Dexterity and Its Development*, translated and published as part of Latash, M. L. and Turvey, M. T. (Eds) *Dexterity and Its Development* (Philadelphia: Lawrence Erlbaum).

Bloom, Benjamin S. (Ed.) (1956) *Taxonomy of Educational Objectives, the Classification of Educational Goals – Handbook I: Cognitive Domain* (New York: McKay) Secondary material is widely available on the Internet, e.g. http://www.coun.uvic.ca/learning/exams/blooms-taxonomy.html (accessed 14 October 2008).

BPS (2007) *The 2007 Annual Report* (Leicester: British Psychological Society) available as http://www.bps.org.uk/the-society/aims-and-objectives/annual-report-and-other-society-docs/annual-report_home.cfm (accessed 9 July 2008).

Bruer, J. T. (1997) 'Education and the Brain: A Bridge Too Far' in *Educational Researcher*, Vol. 26, No. 8, pp. 4–16.

Butterworth, B. (2001) 'What Makes a Prodigy?' in *Nature Neuroscience*, Vol. 4, No. 1, pp. 11–12.

Cosmides, L. and Tooby J. (1997) 'Evolutionary Psychology: A Primer' (Santa Barbara: Center for Evolutionary Psychology) http://www.psych.ucsb.edu/research/cep/primer.html (accessed 27 June 2008).

Dweck, Carol S. (1999) *Self-theories: Their Role in Motivation, Personality and Development* (Philadelphia: Psychology Press).

Flynn, James R. (2007) *What is Intelligence?: Beyond the Flynn Effect* (Cambridge: Cambridge University Press).

Fox, Douglas (2007) 'Remote Control Brains' in *New Scientist*, 21 July 2007, pp. 30–34.

'Go Brain-boosters' (2008) in *New Scientist*, 13 December 2008, p. 6.

Gordon, P., Aldrich, R. and Dean, D. (1991) *Education and Policy in England in the Twentieth Century* (London: Woburn Press).

Greely, H., Sahakian, B., Harris, J., Kessler, R. C., Gazzaniga, M., Campbell, P. and Farah, M. J. (2008) 'Towards Responsible Use of Cognitive-enhancing Drugs by the Healthy' in *Nature*, 11 December 2008, pp. 702–705.

Huang, G. T. (2008) 'Essence of Thought' in *New Scientist*, 31 May 2008, pp. 30–33.

James, J. E., Gregg, M. E., Kane, M., Harte, F. (2005) 'Dietary Caffeine, Performance and Mood: Enhancing and Restorative Effects after Controlling for Withdrawal Reversal' in *Neuropsychobiology*, Vol. 52, No. 1, pp. 1–10.

Jensen, Eric (2008) (2nd Edition) *Brain-based Learning: The New Paradigm of Teaching* (London: Corwin Press).

Keyes, D. (1959) 'Flowers for Algernon' in *Fantasy and Science Fiction* and available at https://www.educ.kent.edu/community/DOCWHIZ/rdng4.html (accessed 24 May 2007).

Latash, M. L. and Turvey, M. T. (Eds) *Dexterity and Its Development* (Philadelphia: Lawrence Erlbaum).

Lynch, Gary (2006) 'Glutamate-based Therapeutic Approaches: Ampakines' in *Current Opinion in Pharmacology*, Vol. 6, No. 1, pp. 82–88.

Maley, J. (2008) 'Changing the Nature of Human Beings' in *Sydney Morning Herald*, 10 August 2008.

Miller, George A. (1956) 'The Magic Number 7 Plus or Minus 2' in *The Psychological Review*, Vol. 63, pp. 81–97 and available at http://www.musanim.com/miller1956 (accessed 24 May 2007).

Morris, E. (2008) 'Teachers in Charge of Change' in *Education Today*, Vol. 58, No. 2, pp. 5–11.

Muller, U., Steffanhagen, N., Regenthal, R. and Bublak, P. (2004) 'Effects of Modafinil on Working Memory Processes in Humans' in *Psychopharmacology*, Vol. 177, pp. 161–169.

Myrick, H., Malcolm, R., Taylor, B. and LaRowe, S. (2004) 'Modafinil: preclinical, clinical, and postmarketing surveillance, a review of abuse liability issues' in *Annals of Clinical Psychiatry*, Vol. 16, pp. 101–109.

Nintendo (2006) 'Dr Kawashima's Brain Training' http://www.braintraining.com.au/training.html (accessed 9 July 2008).

OECD (2007) *Understanding the Brain: The Birth of a Learning Science* (Paris: OECD).

Popper, K. and Eccles, J. C. (1983) *The Self and Its Brain* (London: Routledge).

Postman, Neil (1985) *Amusing Ourselves to Death: Public Discourse in the Age of Show Business* (New York: Penguin).

Randall, D. C., Shneerson, J. M., Plaha, K. K. and File, S. E. (2003) 'Modafinil Affects Mood, but Not Cognitive Function in Healthy Young Volunteers' in *Human Psychopharmacology*, Vol. 18, pp. 163–173.

Rieber, Robert W. (Ed.) (1997) *The Collected Works of L. S. Vygotsky, Volume 4: The History of the Development of Higher Mental Functions* (New York: Plenum Press) (Translated by Marie J. Hall).

Rose, N. (1999) *Governing the Soul* (2nd Edition) (London: Free Association Books).

Shallice, Tim (1988) *From Neuropsychology to Mental Structure* (Cambridge: Cambridge University Press).

Smith, Alistair (2004) (Revised Edition) *The Brain's Behind It* (Stafford: Network Educational Press).

Springer, S. P. and Deutsch, G. (1985) *Left Brain, Right Brain* (New York: W. H. Freeman and Company).

Sweller, J., van Merriënboer, J. J. G., and Paas, F. (1998) 'Cognitive Architecture and Instructional Design' in *Educational Psychology Review*, Vol. 10, pp. 251–296.

TLRP (2007) *Neuroscience and Education: Issues and Opportunities* (London: TLRP) and available from http://www.tlrp.org/pub/commentaries.html (accessed 27 May 2009).

Tomlinson, Stephen (2005) *Head Masters: Phrenology, Secular Education, and Nineteenth-Century Social Thought* (Tuscaloosa: University of Alabama Press).

Turner, D. A. (2004) *Theory of Education* (London: Continuum).

—(2007) *Theory and Practice of Education* (London: Continuum).

Turner, D. C., Robbins, T. W., Clark, L., Aron, A. R., Dowson, J. and Sahakian, B. J. (2003) 'Cognitive Enhancing Effects of Modafinil in Healthy Volunteers' in *Psychopharmacology*, Vol. 165, pp. 260–269.

Turner, D. C., Clark, L., Dowson, J., Robbins, T. W. and Sahakian, B. J. (2004a) 'Modafinil Improves Cognition and Response Inhibition in Adult ADHD' in *Biological Psychiatry*, Vol. 55, pp. 1031–1039.

Turner, D. C., Clark, L., Pomarol-Clotet, E., McKenna, P., Robbins, T. W. and Sahakian, B. J. (2004b) 'Modafinil Improves Cognition and Attentional Set Shifting in Patients with Chronic Schizophrenia' in *Neuropsychopharmacology*, Vol. 29, pp. 1363–1373.

Tysome, Tony (2007) 'Pills Provide Brain Boost for Academics' in the *Times Higher Education Supplement*, pp. 6–7.

Weisberg, D. S., Keil, F. C., Goodstein, J., Rawson, E. and Gray, J. R. (2008) 'The Seductive Allure of Neuroscience Explanations' in *Journal of Cognitive Neuroscience*, Vol. 20, No. 3, pp. 470–477.

Index